Contemporary Theorists for Medical Sociology

'A well-crafted account of the work of several contemporary theorists in sociology in relation to their relevance for medical sociology. It has the potential to be highly influential in stimulating new insights and uses of the work of theorists sometimes overlooked in medical sociology.'

William C. Cockerham, Distinguished Professor of Sociology,
University of Alabama at Birmingham, USA

Contemporary Theorists for Medical Sociology explores the work of key social theorists and the application of their ideas to issues around health and illness.

Encouraging students and researchers to use mainstream sociological thought to inform and deepen their knowledge and understanding of the many arenas of health and healthcare, this text discusses and critically reviews the work of several influential contemporary thinkers, including Foucault, Bauman, Habermas, Luhmann, Bourdieu, Merleau-Ponty, Wallerstein, Archer, Deleuze, Guattari, and Castells.

Each chapter includes a critical introduction to the central theses of a major social theorist, ways in which their ideas might inform medical sociology and some worked examples of how their ideas can be applied. Containing contributions from established scholars, rising stars, and innovative practitioners, this book is a valuable read for those studying and researching the sociology of health and illness.

Graham Scambler is Professor of Medical Sociology at University College London, UK.

Critical Studies in Health and Society
Series Editors: Simon J. Williams & Gillian Bendelow

This major new international book series takes a critical look at health in a rapidly changing social world. The series includes theoretically sophisticated and empirically informed contributions on cutting-edge issues from leading figures within the sociology of health and allied disciplines and domains. Other titles in the series include:

Medical Technologies and the Life World
The social construction of normality
Edited by Sonia Olin Lauritzen and Lars-Christer Hyden

Women's Health and Social Change
Ellen Annandale

Contesting Psychiatry
Social movements in mental health
Nick Crossley

Lifestyle in Medicine
Gary Easthope and Emily Hansen

Medical Sociology and Old Age
Towards a sociology of health in later life
Paul Higgs and Ian Rees Jones

Emotional Labour in Health Care
The Unmanaged Heart of Nursing
Catherine Theodosius

Globalisation, Markets and Healthcare Policy
Redrawing the Patient as Consumer
Jonathan Tritter, Meri Koivusalo and Eeva Ollila

Written in a lively, accessible and engaging style, with many thought-provoking insights, the series will cater to a truly interdisciplinary audience of researchers, professionals, practitioners and policy makers with an interest in health and social change.

Those interested in submitting proposals for single or co-authored, edited or co-edited volumes should contact the series editors, Simon J. Williams (s.j.williams@warwick.ac.uk) and Gillian Bendelow (g.a.bendelow@sussex.ac.uk).

Contemporary Theorists for Medical Sociology

Edited by Graham Scambler

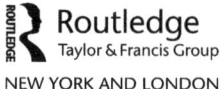

NEW YORK AND LONDON

First published 2012
by Routledge
2 Park Square, Milton Park, Abingdon, Oxon OX14 4RN

Simultaneously published in the USA and Canada
by Routledge
711 Third Avenue, New York, NY 10017

Routledge is an imprint of the Taylor & Francis Group, an informa business

© 2012 selection and editorial material, Graham Scambler;
individual chapters, the contributors

The right of the editor to be identified as the author of the editorial
material, and of the chapter authors for their individual contributions,
has been asserted by them in accordance with sections 77 and 78 of the
Copyright, Designs and Patents Act 1988.

All rights reserved. No part of this book may be reprinted or reproduced or
utilised in any form or by any electronic, mechanical, or other means, now
known or hereafter invented, including photocopying and recording, or in any
information storage or retrieval system, without permission in writing from the
publishers.

Trademark notice: Product or corporate names may be trademarks or registered
trademarks, and are used only for identification and explanation without
intent to infringe.

British Library Cataloguing in Publication Data
A catalogue record for this book is available from the British Library

Library of Congress Cataloging-in-Publication Data
Contemporary theorists for medical sociology / edited by Graham Scambler.
p. cm. -- (Critical studies in health and society)
1. Social medicine. 2. Public welfare. 3. Sociology--Philosophy.
I. Scambler, Graham.
RA418.C6723 2013
362.1--dc23
2011041146

ISBN13: 978-0-415-59782-1 (hbk)
ISBN13: 978-0-415-59783-8 (pbk)
ISBN13: 978-0-203-12268-6 (ebk)

Typeset in Baskerville by
Taylor & Francis Books

Contents

	List of illustrations	vii
	List of contributors	viii
	Introduction: theory, theorists and the sociology of health GRAHAM SCAMBLER	1
1	Foucault, health and healthcare ALAN PETERSEN	7
2	Consuming bodies: Zygmunt Bauman on the difference between fitness and health PAUL HIGGS	20
3	Jürgen Habermas: politics and morality in health and medicine GEMMA EDWARDS	33
4	Luhmann's social systems theory, health and illness BARRY GIBSON AND OLGA BOIKO	49
5	Bourdieu and the impact of health and illness in the lifeworld SASHA SCAMBLER	71
6	Merleau-Ponty, medicine and the body NICK CROSSLEY	87
7	World systems theory and the epidemiological transition MARTIN HYDE AND ANTHONY ROSIE	104
8	Archer, morphogenesis and the role of agency in the sociology of health inequalities GRAHAM SCAMBLER	131

9	Deleuze and Guattari NICK J. FOX	150
10	Health and medicine in the information age: Castells, informational capitalism and the network society SIMON J. WILLIAMS	167
	Index	193

Illustrations

Figures

4.1	The use of distinctions in Luhmann's social systems theory	52
7.1	Spatial boundaries of world-system networks	119
7.2	Adult mortality rate (per 100,000) by export concentration index: 2008	122
7.3	Under fives mortality rate (per 100,000) by export concentration index: 2009	123
7.4	Proportion of deaths due to communicable, maternal, perinatal and nutritional conditions by export concentration index: 2004	124
8.1	The three-stage model	137
8.2	The theory so far	141

Tables

4.1	Luhmann's analytical strategies	56
7.1	The classic (Western) model	108
8.1	Modes of reflexivity	137

Contributors

Olga Boiko is Associate Research Fellow at the Institute of Health Services Research, Peninsula College of Medicine and Dentistry, University of Exeter. Olga has been working on the social systems theory of Niklas Luhmann since completing her PhD at the University of Sheffield in 2009; in particular she has been working on its applications to the analysis of healthcare communication in dentistry (Boiko *et al.* [2011] 'Form and semantics of communication in dental encounters: oral health, probability and time', *Sociology of Health and Illness*, 33(1): 16–32). The dentine sensitivity study that features in this volume is a subsequent contribution that demonstrates a growing potential of this meta-theory to medical sociology. Her current research continues to be informed by systems theory and a realistic evaluation framework in exploring academia–NHS collaborations in the South West of England.

Nick Crossley is a professor in sociology at the University of Manchester. His most recent book, *Towards Relational Sociology* (Routledge 2011), argues for a form of sociology centred upon the analysis of interaction, networks and social relations. He has recently finished two empirical projects, one on campus-based political networks (with Joseph Ibrahim) and the other on 'covert networks' (with Rachel Stevenson, Gemma Edwards and Ellie Harries). In addition to writing these projects up he is now working on an analysis of the network structures of the punk and post-punk musical 'worlds' of Manchester, London, Liverpool and Sheffield between 1976 and 1980.

Gemma Edwards is Lecturer in Sociology at the University of Manchester, UK. Her main interests are in applied critical theory and social movements. She has written on Habermas's New Social Movement Theory and has applied ideas of colonization and resistance to the UK public sector and trade unions. Her other research interests include social networks and participation in militant activism, with a methodological interest in mixed-method social network analysis. She has a forthcoming book, *Social Movements and Protest*.

Nick J. Fox is honorary Professor of Sociology at the University of Sheffield, in the School of Health and Related Research. He is the author of books and articles on a range of topics concerning social theory, health and technology, with recent work on health assemblages, health identities, and the pharmaceuticalisation of life. His most recent book, entitled *The Body*, was published by Polity Press in 2012.

Barry Gibson is Senior Lecturer in Medical Sociology at the University of Sheffield. His research interests include exploring the experience of oral health conditions such as dentine sensitivity and dry mouth. His long-term projects include developing a sociology of the mouth in everyday life. This work involves the use of Niklas Luhmann's systems theory, consumerism and the sociology of the body.

Paul Higgs is Professor of the Sociology of Ageing at University College London where he teaches medical sociology. He is co-editor of the journal *Social Theory and Health* and is the author (with Chris Gilleard) of *Cultures of Ageing: Self, Citizen and the Body* (2000) and *Contexts of Ageing: Class, Cohort and Community* (2005). He is also the co-author of *Medical Sociology and Old Age* (2009) and *Ageing in a Consumer Society* (2008) and co-edited *Consumption and Generational Change* (2009). Professor Higgs' research interests include the Third Age; embodiment; identity; generations, cohorts and ageing; and consumption and later life. He is a collaborator on the English Longitudinal Study of Ageing (ELSA). Paul Higgs has published extensively in the fields of social gerontology and medical sociology. He is currently co-authoring a book on the embodiment of ageing and jointly editing a volume on social class and later life.

Martin Hyde is Senior Researcher at the Stress Research Institute at Stockholm University. He has worked on a number of large cross-national surveys of ageing and later life including the English Longitudinal Study of Ageing (ELSA) and the Survey of Health, Ageing and Retirement in Europe (SHARE). His research interests are the changing nature of later life, the impact of labour market exit on health and well-being, cross-national research and the impact of globalization on health. He has published a number of papers and book chapters on these issues as well as co-authoring *Ageing in a Consumer Society: From Passive to Active Consumption in Britain*.

Alan Petersen is Professor of Sociology, School of Political and Social Inquiry, Monash University in Melbourne, Australia. Alan has published extensively in the sociology of health and medicine, and science and technology studies. In his work he has drawn extensively (although not exclusively) on the work of Michel Foucault and his followers. His most recent books are *The Politics of Bioethics* (Routledge, 2011), *The Body in Question: A Socio-Cultural Approach* (Routledge, 2007), and *Nanotechnologies, Risk and Communication* (Palgrave, 2009) (with Alison Anderson, Stuart Allan and Clare Wilkinson). He is currently working on an edited book, *Aging Men: Masculinities and Modern Medicine* (Routledge, forthcoming 2012) (with Antje Kampf and Barbara Marshall) and a sole-authored book, *Hope in Health: The Socio-Politics of Expectations* (Palgrave, 2013).

Anthony Rosie has taught social theory and historical–comparative sociology at Sheffield Hallam University since 1995. He began his career teaching English in secondary schools, worked as a youth and community work trainer and has regularly taught both sociology and teacher education. Most recently he has been tutor for PhD programmes in social science at Sheffield Hallam. He was awarded a national teaching fellowship in 2001, a senior fellowship of the Higher Education Academy in 2007. He was Director of the HEA subject centre for sociology, anthropology and politics from 2003 to 2005 and has also been a director of a HEFCE centre for excellence in learning and teaching. He has served on national committees for learning and teaching and is editor of *Enhancing Learning in the Social Sciences*. He is currently emeritus professor of social science education.

Graham Scambler is Professor of Medical Sociology at UCL. He has written widely on issues of social and critical theory, health, chronic and disabling conditions, health inequalities, sex work and sport. His most recent book is *New Directions in the Sociology of Chronic and Disabling Conditions* (co-edited with Sasha Scambler), published by Palgrave Macmillan in 2010. He is currently co-authoring books on *Long-term Conditions* and *Health Inequalities* for Polity Press, and *Sport in a Changing Society* for Palgrave Macmillan. He is founding co-editor of the international journal *Social Theory and Health*.

Sasha Scambler is Lecturer in Sociology at King's College London Dental Institute. She has carried out extensive work on the experiences of families with Batten disease and researched and published on the application of disability and social theory to chronic disabling conditions and loneliness in later life. Sasha is co-editor of the journal *Social Science and Dentistry* and has published two books, including a co-edited collection *New Directions in the Sociology of Chronic and Disabling Conditions*, which brings together leading international researchers in medical sociology and disability theory to critically review the sociological approach to chronic and disabling conditions.

Simon J. Williams is a professor of sociology at the University of Warwick. He has published extensively in the sociology of health, medicine, the body and emotion over the years. This work has in turn been augmented through more recent biopolitical interests, particularly the power and prospects of the neurosciences today and in the near future. His latest book is *The Politics of Sleep: Governing (Un)Consciousness in the Late Modern Age* (2011, Palgrave Macmillan).

Introduction
Theory, theorists and the sociology of health

Graham Scambler

There is a sense in which medical sociology, indeed all sociology, is necessarily a theoretical project. It can neither begin nor end in a social vacuum: we are products of our times and places. Moreover to assent to any one proposition about social phenomena is to dissent from others; and to assent is to sign up wittingly or otherwise to a particular way of seeing or presenting the social world within which we are all actors and agents. Sociologists' degree of reflexivity about their theoretical baggage or commitment is variable. When not actually in denial, the positivist is often non-reflexive. For a vast array of non- or post-positivists, however, the theoretical nature of the medical sociological project is incontrovertible, a matter for open conjecture and evidence-based debate.

In the introduction to a collection entitled 'Sociological Theory and Medical Sociology' published in 1987 I echoed what was at the time a popular lament, namely that medical sociology remained largely detached from mainstream sociological and social theory. I did not mean by this either that medical sociology was merely positivistic or that it had no history of reflexive theoretical engagement. Such assertions would have been manifestly false. My point was that there seemed particularly scant interest in those theories that ranged from macro- through meso- to micro-phenomena in the health domain, *theories that linked societal order and change with everyday thoughts and behaviour.* Once the heady early days of (structurally oriented) Parsonian structural functionalism versus (agency-oriented) symbolic interactionism were over, medical sociology's more pluralistic or 'multi-paradigmatic' ambitions seemed to wane. It was as if medical sociologists in North America, Europe, and Australasia aspired, at best, to theories of Merton's middle range. Most hostility was directed towards one of Wright Mills' (1963) two perils, 'abstracted empiricism', there being little evidence of any post-Parsonian predilection for 'grand theory'. A lack of 'sociological imagination' appeared self-evident. There also seemed to be a lot of positivist research about.

On the whole it is a judgement I stand by, albeit with a qualification or two. It is questionable, for example, whether I made sufficient allowance for my own background and interpretation of events as a philosophically trained sociologist. I may have been too readily seduced by macro-theory, or even, in unguarded moments, by grand theory. As a medical sociologist closeted and isolated in a series of London University Medical Schools I may also have been overexposed to abstracted empiricism. Moreover there was more going on than perhaps I appreciated, especially in mainstream sociology departments in the US, where there was growing acknowledgement and application to health of schools of thought and perspectives outside of functionalism and interactionism, including systems theory, critical theory, rational choice theory, and so on (Cockerham, 2000; Cockerham & Scambler, 2010).

But how do things stand nearly a quarter of a century after? It makes sense to introduce what is in many ways a revisiting of territory some of us felt we needed visas to enter in 1987 via a brief reconsideration of the role of theory in medical sociology, or the sociology of health and illness. Accomplishment and tensions are both apparent. There is clear evidence of greater reflexivity and of more and increasingly sophisticated dialogues between social and sociological theorists and 'specialists' committed to understanding and/or explaining behaviours around health, illness and healthcare (de Maio, 2010). Some of these dialogues are explicitly theoretical, others implicitly so. The former seek to knowingly apply, develop, or innovate around theories whose origins and foci lie outside of the health domain, while the latter are more fortuitously indebted to this same body of work. For example, the work of Parsons and Merton survive respectively in the systems–theoretical perspectives of Luhmann and in the theories of the middle-range that characterize much of contemporary professional medical sociological enquiry. Interactionism too remains a vital ingredient of the sub-discipline: much of the continuing research on chronic illness is premised on the work of Mead, via Bulmer, Roth, Glaser and Strauss, and others. The genius of Foucault has proved inspirational, principally via assorted, strong versus weak species of social constructionism. Conflict theory born of Marx and developed by the critical theorists of the Frankfurt School (among others) has also informed select branches of medical sociology. Bourdieu has his advocates, as have feminist and neo-colonialist thinkers and the critical realism inspired by Bhaskar's challenge to orthodox scientific enquiry.

Against this narrative of steady, growing accomplishment should be set novel institutional pressures on occupationally insecure medical sociologists to be circumscribed or 'cost-effective', that is, one way or another to underwrite their salaries. Social and sociological theorists tend not to raise money through research and can find themselves under pressure to justify their posts 'in difficult times'. There is evidence too of a related 'McDonaldization' of (medical) sociology, an often counter-productive emphasis on uniformity in the delivery and assessment of disciplinary products. Journal impact factors prevail, and peer-reviewed articles have typically to comply with strict parameters of format, length, and even orthodoxy. Appraisals of work and worth must be quantified (Ritzer, 2001; Scambler, 2005). There is a threat of theoretical 'taming' here (Scambler, 1996).

Paradoxically, in the immediate aftermath of the 2008/2009 'global financial crisis', which is witnessing an aggressive rearguard action on the part of neo-liberalism's beneficiaries and a predictably virulent pro-workfare anti-welfarism, an urgent need for theoretical engagement coincides with heavy constraints on its delivery. In my view, theoreticians' contributions to 'critical', and even more, 'public' medical sociology are as vital now as they are personally challenging to deliver (Burawoy, 2005).

So it is perhaps an appropriate juncture to nourish an explicit, theory-oriented medical sociology. But adopting the same format as in 1987 requires additional justification: it is not axiomatic that selecting noted theorists and either underwriting or positing their salience for professional and policy medical sociology is an optimal device. Maybe, however, it is a useful *heuristic* device. In its predecessor, 'Sociological Theory and Medical Sociology', the theorists picked as a result of a dialogue between editor and contributor, were: Marx (David Blane), Durkheim (Steven Taylor and Clive Ashworth), Parsons (Uta Gerhardt), Foucault (David Armstrong), Freud (Karl Figlio), Goffman (Simon Williams), Habermas (Graham Scambler), Weber (Sheila Hillier), and Offe (Ray Fitzpatrick). An equivalent dialogue this time round has led to the inclusion of: Foucault (Alan Peterson), Bauman (Paul Higgs), Habermas (Susan Edwards), Luhmann (Barry Gibson and Olga Boiko), Bourdieu (Sasha Scambler), Merleau-Ponty (Nick Crossley), Wallerstein (Martin Hyde and Anthony Rosie), Archer (Graham Scambler), Deleueze and Guatteri (Nick Fox), and Castells (Simon Williams). The second appearance of Foucault, a continuing major influence on medical sociology internationally, requires little defence, while that of Habermas draws in a new and subtle commentator. The remaining contributions, I suggest, speak for themselves, although a case could undoubtedly have been made for a dozen other theorists.

It is doubtful if there are more informed, perspicacious and engaged commentators on Foucault's relevance for understanding health and healthcare than Alan Petersen. He opens this collection with a sharp, fair-minded yet critical review of Foucault's work, charting his input into theory and research in the multiple arenas of health whilst also pointing out his silence on others. He locates him as a key twentieth-century social theorist before surveying the role and reach of later Foucauldian scholarship in enriching our grasp of the health 'field'. But there is a critical edge to his exposition and evaluation: there are 'blind spots' in Foucault's work. There are problems issuing from the 'vagueness' of Foucauldian terminology; he under-theorized group agency, contestation, and counter-discourse; and he was 'inattentive' to political economy and what might be called the structures of class, gender, ethnicity, and so on. To take Foucault at his own evaluation, he suggests, is to adopt his work as a 'toolbox of ideas', and it is an orientation Petersen continues to find rewarding.

Paul Higgs dips into the striking insights to be found in Zygmunt Bauman's ever-expanding body of work to emerge with a distinction between 'fitness' and 'health'. He maintains that this is especially salient for a credible theory of embodiment in contemporary consumer society. Fitness is not for Bauman an extension of health but a going beyond or transcendence of it. He points to a new relationship between illness, health, and fitness. It is one that challenges the conventional dichotomy between 'normal' and 'abnormal' by emphasizing the 'unrealisable demands of fitness'. A complex and subtle case is made that the preoccupation with survival characteristic of producer society has been succeeded by a preoccupation with quality of life in consumer society; and that it is in this context that the desire for fitness has emerged as the light at the end of a tunnel of indeterminate length.

Habermas, like Foucault, featured in 'Sociological Theory and Medical Sociology'. Gemma Edwards affirms the relevance of his theory of society and social action for health and healthcare in her contribution. She offers an eloquent summary of his theory of communicative action, focusing on the complex social differentiation of modern societies and the 'de-coupling' of system and lifeworld. Extending her own previous work, she rehearses and critiques Habermas' system/lifeworld distinction. It makes little sense, she argues, to allocate a healthcare service to *either* system *or* lifeworld. System and lifeworld are best seen as two different ways of doing things – two logics of action – that exist *everywhere*. Health movements in the past have agitated for *more* not less state engagement. Embodied health movements in the present, however, are principally significant because they compel consideration of how questions of health and healthcare are, 'first and foremost, questions about politics and morality'.

Luhmann's work is notoriously resistant to summary, and because of this critiques of his social systems theory can seem unduly arcane and esoteric. Barry Gibson and Olga Boiko grasp the nettle. They offer a succinct account of Luhmann's narrative of modernity, showing how systematic communications eventually specialize to the point where systems 'separate or differentiate themselves'. This results in self-referentiality or 'autopoiesis'. Autopoietic systems have their own dynamics: they are organizationally 'closed' but energetically 'open'. They then document how this 'high-level' theoretical orientation has been of service to the fields of health and illness. They close their chapter with an account of how Luhmann's work might inform mundane everyday events like patterns of communication about dentine sensitivity.

Bourdieu's contributions to social theory have been a strong if intermittent resource for medical sociology. Sasha Scambler acknowledges this in her general exposition. She explicates core concepts – 'field', 'capital', 'habitus', 'bodily hexis' – prior to showing how these might help frame sociological accounts of the impact of chronic and disabling conditions on the lifeworld. She does this through a detailed and research-based consideration of how (typically young) people face a foreshortened life with Batten disease. Crucially this experience occurs in the intimate company of their parents/families and/or significant others, who summon up and put to use the various forms of capital at their disposal. It is a poignant as well as a suggestive sociological narrative. It is also a narrative that favours further integration between sociological and disability theory (Scambler & Scambler, 2010).

Nick Crossley's chapter on Merleau-Ponty may be a less obvious source of sociological inspiration, at least to those under a certain age. To others the latter's 'Phenomenology of Perception' and 'The Structure of Behaviour' are under-utilized texts. Merleau-Ponty is presented here as a significant philosopher of embodiment. The chapter offers a succinct summary of this philosophy before discussing the challenges it represents to orthodox (Cartesian) conceptualizations of the 'medical body': it is a philosophy favouring constructionist and holist approaches, but with qualifications. When we fall ill, our bodies cease to be 'blind spots' for us: they become available for objectification and observation. The final paragraphs, however, move on from the ramifications of the lived bodies of people-as-patients to raise intriguing questions about the embodiment of medical practice itself.

Wallerstein's world system theory transports a Marxist orientation to modernity beyond the nation-state and insists on an engagement with historical and comparative research. The importance of the astonishingly wide-ranging and influential research of the French historian Braudel is noted. After briefly reviewing world systems theory, Martin Hyde and Anthony Rosie ask how world systems theory might inform and – sociologically speaking – invigorate 'epidemiological transition theory'. Epidemiological transition theory is introduced and critiqued. The authors suggest that while epidemiological transition theory affords a serviceable framework for examining changes in the health of a population, it neglects interconnections between states and the impact these have on the epidemiological transition. Population health, they contend, is 'relational', insofar as the factors that determine it are part of the world system. To buttress their case they deploy a mix of data on trade and mortality, focusing on the region of West Africa to illustrate their argument.

Margaret Archer's writings are unlikely to be known by medical sociologists. She is most eminent as a theorist and a sociologist of education. She is my theorist of choice in this volume: she has over the years proved a subtle, shrewd and independent-minded disciple of a (critical) realist orientation to sociological research and practice. The focus here is on her recent work on those 'internal conversations' we all recognize and count as integral to our humanity. I mount a case that the wealthy and powerful in our society, neglected causal progenitors of health inequalities in the UK and elsewhere, display a socially structured, if not structurally determined, cast of mind. Drawing on Archer's analysis, they comprise an ideal type of 'focused autonomous reflexives'. A broader thesis is that medical sociology has paid insufficient attention to the socially structured mindsets and predispositions of key actors in the field of health inequalities.

The chapter committed to the theories of Deleuze and Guattari and authored by Nick Fox also focuses on the body. It is essential, he insists, that sociologists of health, illness, and medicine come to terms with the dual – biological and social – character of the body. Deleuze and Guattari's analyses are premised on a link between body, subjectivity, and culture. An eloquent, select exposition of these analyses follows. The concept of the 'body *with* organs' is introduced, together with those of its 'de-' and 're-territorialization'. Deleuze and Guattari align themselves with the de-territorialization of, or resistance to, the body-with-organs, which gives rise to the notion of (a process of) 'nomadology' as a strategy for living. It is a model that is here applied as well as announced. At this point the 'body *without* organs' features: this denotes the limit of what a body can do in terms of its relations and the 'play of forces' of those relations. Embodiment is not the passive outcome but a dynamic and reflexive 'reading' of the social by an active, motivated human being.

The final chapter by Simon Williams takes the influential sociologist Castells as his point of departure. This is a notably original piece of work in that only rarely have medical sociologists drawn, even circuitously, on Castells' framing of the network society to better describe and/or explain phenomena of health, illness, or healthcare. Considerable potential is discerned in Castells' deepening of his analysis via the idea of communicative power. The unfolding of his published work is reflected. At the core of the argument is the idea that Castells is important because his theories offer: (a) key theories relating to the dynamics of the information age (embracing global complexity, networks, flows, mobilities, and so on), and (b) resources for a 'renewal' of (medical) sociology. Illustrations in support of this case are offered for continuing discussion.

This book, in the vein of its predecessor, will have served its purpose if it acts as a catalyst, provoking or tempting medical sociologists, students, and others interested in the multiple arenas of health to turn expectantly to established and challenging bodies of social and sociological theory to frame or deepen their research or understanding. It may be a less urgent project than in the Thatcherite mid 1980s: medical sociology is a more sophisticated sub-discipline now than it was then, at least in the UK. But on the other hand, in the 'new England' of a neo-Thatcherite, Cameron-led 'coalition' committed to the re-commodification of all things health related, including the National Health Service, maybe not. In any case, and independently of one's (Weberian) *value reference*, the call for reflexivity and theory remains undiminished.

References

Burawoy, T. (2005) For public sociology. *American Sociological Review* 70: 4–28.
Cockerham, W. (2000) Medical sociology at the millennium. In Eds Quah, S. & Sales, A. *The International Handbook of Sociology*. London: Sage.
Cockerham, W. & Scambler, G. (2010) Medical sociology and sociological theory. In Ed Cockerham, W. *The Blackwell Companion to Medical Sociology*. Oxford: Blackwell.
Di Maio, F. (2010) Health and Social Theory. London: Palgrave Macmillan.
Ritzer, G. (2001) The McDonaldization of American sociology: a metasociological analysis. In Ritzer, G. Explorations in Social Theory: from Metatheorizing to Rationalization. London: Sage.
Scambler, G. (1996) The 'project of modernity' and the parameters for a critical sociology: an argument with illustrations from medical sociology. *Sociology* 30: 567–981.
——(1987) Introduction. In Ed Scambler, G: Medical Sociology and Sociological Theory. London: Tavistock.
——(2005) General introduction: medical sociology: past, present and future. In Ed Scambler, G. (ed.): *Medical Sociology: Major Themes in Health and Social Welfare*. Volume 1: The Nature of Medical Sociology. London: Routledge.
Scambler, G. & Scambler, S. (eds) (2010) *New Directions in the Sociology of Chronic and Disabling Conditions: Assaults on the Lifeworld*. London: Palgrave Macmillan.
Wright Mills, C. (1963) *The Sociological Imagination*. Harmondsworth: Penguin.

1 Foucault, health and healthcare

Alan Petersen

Of the many social scientists who have contributed to the field of health and healthcare, few have shaped thought to the extent that the French philosopher and historian Michel Foucault (1926–83) has. Foucault's work has been influential internationally not only because he wrote specifically about health and medicine, but because his work, which traversed many topics (such as the history of crime and punishment, sexuality, and the formation of knowledge), offered a rich 'toolkit' of ideas that may be taken up and applied in understanding diverse issues within the arena of health and healthcare; for example, responses to disability, practices of body modification, the impacts of new biomedical technologies, the practices of dentistry. The 'Foucault effect' is evident in many disciplines or fields of study that touch on questions of health, including sociology, anthropology, social policy, business and marketing, medical education and communication studies. This effect can be explained by the fact that Foucault offered critical perspectives on matters of wide concern, both challenging taken-for-granted ways of understanding and offering a new agenda for research and policy. Foucault's legacy is difficult to neatly summarise since it informs the work of many writers to varying degrees, and not always explicitly. This chapter examines some of the key concepts developed by Foucault and how these have been and may be applied by researchers in the fields of health and healthcare. To begin, it is important to understand the kind of theorist that Foucault was and how his way of thinking differed from, say, Marxists or theorists of modernity. All writers are products of their time, generating work that reflects the preoccupations and values of their society and, although he was a critical thinker, like other writers, Foucault had his biases and 'blind spots', which we need to recognise.

Foucault as a theorist

Foucault has been described variously as a structuralist, a poststructuralist and a postmodern theorist. While this perhaps reflects the absence of definitional clarity among writers, it also reveals much about the character of Foucault's work, which defies easy definition. His work engaged with and is in many senses consistent with more established traditions of thought and yet also offers new perspectives on phenomena such as medicine and crime and punishment. His historical approach, described as genealogy, offers a 'history of the present', focusing on discontinuity rather than continuity, which is a feature of much historiography, with the aim of disrupting our taken-for-granted ways of knowing and showing that our ways of thinking and acting could be different. While conventional history seeks to confirm the present by offering a linear account of events, with an assumed pattern of causation (i.e. teleological) implying progress and an inevitability of outcomes, genealogy seeks to disrupt our conceptions of the present, by drawing attention to how these are reliant on shifting discourses and practices linked to particular operations of power. Foucault understood discourse as a collection of related statements and events, which are a historical manifestation of a particular configuration of knowledge and power. (He used the shorthand 'power-knowledge' to indicate this inextricable relationship.) His book, *Discipline and Punish* (1977), for example, documented the discursive shift in the mechanisms of power corresponding with the rise of the modern period, commencing in the eighteenth century, whereby so-called sovereign power, which resides with the king and is manifest in the public execution, is gradually replaced by disciplinary power, which involves a more dispersed form of power involving control over the body and mind through specialised institutions such as schools, prisons, workplaces and hospitals. In this book, he identifies the panopticon, an architectural design developed by the utilitarian Jeremy Bentham for controlling prisoners, as the archetypal modern form of power. This operates on the principle that individuals can be incited to govern themselves, rather than be governed by an external agency, through specific techniques, such as the design of buildings and the monitoring of public spaces. In the contemporary period, surveillance cameras erected in public spaces arguably adopt this principle, the assumption being that people will police themselves if they never know whether or not they are under surveillance.

In seeking to characterise Foucault's work, it is common for writers to distinguish between the 'early' and 'later' Foucault. The former is seen to focus on 'techniques of domination', particularly mechanisms of regulation and surveillance, while the latter is seen to emphasise 'techniques of the self', which draws attention to the ways in which individuals regulate or 'govern' themselves. However, although the topics and emphases in Foucault's work changed over time – as it does with all writers – it is possible to see some recurring themes in his writing. For example, his early work on surveillance finds expression in his later work on 'governance of the self' (see below), which involves surveillance of one's own actions and thoughts. Further, aspects of his early writing (in *The Birth of the Clinic* [1975]) on the discourse of 'the body', which shapes the way the material body is seen, described and acted upon (particularly through scientific medicine), finds resonance in his later three-volume work on the history of sexuality, particularly Volume One, where he describes the operations of 'bio-power', the politics of life itself (Foucault, 1980). Notwithstanding these enduring themes, it is evident that in his later work, and particularly in Volumes Two and Three of *The History of Sexuality*, Foucault began to give more attention to the intersection between the 'techniques of domination' and the 'techniques of the self'. These volumes, *The Use of Pleasure* (1987) and *The Care of the Self* (1990), can be seen as an attempt by

Foucault to overcome some early criticisms that he inadequately acknowledged agency and self-determination. The concept he developed, 'technologies of the self' or 'practices of the self', refers to the practices and techniques through which individuals actively fashion their own identities. His work on governmentality, articulated in a series of lectures in his later life, and further developed by writers such as Nicholas Rose (1999) and Mitchell Dean (1999), focuses in particular on the forms of self-governance associated with rule in advanced liberal (or neo-liberal) societies.

While Foucault's work focuses largely on modern society – that is, the period from the eighteenth century – and on the West (with a strong focus on French society), increasingly his work has been taken up and applied to different societies in different periods. For example, his concepts have been applied in studies of Australian indigenous society, to explore how issues of governance operate in the control of subject populations (e.g. Rowse, 1998). Although his work is located in the modern period, Foucault offers a different approach to modern society from sociologists of modernity such as Anthony Giddens, Ulrich Beck and Zygmunt Bauman, who tend to ascribe autonomy to the human subject and to emphasise individual agency and rational action, which Foucault took issue with. Giddens' work, for example, has focused on the choices confronting the individual who is obliged to navigate the multiple risks and opportunities that characterise modern societies (e.g. Giddens, 1991). Foucault's work also differs from Marxists who draw attention to how material conditions and associated class relations shape history. Indeed, Foucault's work grows out of a reaction to a particular, determinist version of Marxism that ascribes an independent force to the economy and the dynamics of class relations. Although he was interested in issues of politics and power, Foucault was inattentive to political economy, which is arguably one 'blind spot' and shortcoming of his work in understanding the operations of modern societies (see below).

What then have been the specific contributions of Foucault to the field of health and healthcare? And how have his ideas been applied by others thus far? In the following paragraphs I outline some major contributions, and indicate further areas where his ideas may be usefully applied. I then conclude by drawing attention to some limitations of Foucault's work and related scholarship, with some suggestions as to how these could be addressed.

The body

Foucault's writing on the body has been without doubt one of his major contributions to health and healthcare, and to social science more generally. A growing focus on the body in sociology and other social sciences in the early 1990s onwards owes much to the growing influence of Foucault during this period. The launch of a new journal, *The Body & Society*, edited by Mike Featherstone and Bryan Turner, two well-known sociologists, who themselves have published widely in this field, signalled a burgeoning interest in social studies of the body that continues in the early 2000s. Much of this has drawn on Foucault's concepts. The growing attention to new biomedical technologies focusing on the modification and surveillance of the body, including genetic testing and treatments, the growing use of MRIs (magnetic resonance imaging), xeno-transplantation (i.e. animal-to-human tissue replacement) and technologies of enhancement (e.g. cosmetic surgery, body piercing, body sculpting, weight-loss products) has called for new theoretical approaches. Foucault's attention to power-knowledge and to the surveillance implications of biomedical practices has inspired writers working on various topics, such as technologies of reproduction, cosmetic surgery and genetic testing. Foucault's work provides something of an antidote to biomedical imperialism, whereby 'health' is viewed as an innate or natural quality of the body, reducible to, for example, genetic makeup, hormones or brain wiring. In particular, Foucault offered tools for exploring the power relations and implications of the 'medical gaze' (see below).

The value of Foucault's work on the body is perhaps nowhere more evident than in the analysis of gender and health. Feminist writers such as Jana Sawicki (*Disciplining Foucault*, 1991) have emphasised the productive power of new technologies of reproduction; that is, the potential for innovations to create categories of human subject, shape subjectivities and give rise to new sites for intervention. As Sawicki argues, rather than viewing such technologies as instruments of oppression – as a means by which men gain increasing control over women's bodies – which early feminists such as Gena Corea (*The Mother Machine*, 1985) argued – such technologies create multiple opportunities for being and action, including resistance. While Foucault himself has been criticised for failing to position himself on questions of gender-based oppression (Barrett, 1991: 151–52; Flax, 1990: 212), his concepts have been extensively employed by feminists who critique the 'essentialist' and universalising tendencies of certain schools of feminist thought. His work has proved especially useful for analysing and bringing a new, nuanced understanding to the experience of managing conditions that entirely or disproportionally affect women, such as menopause, anorexia and endometriosis (e.g. Robertson, 1992; Murtagh, 2003; Seear, 2009). The governmentality perspective has proved especially valuable in highlighting how the self-management of such conditions involves a certain relationship to one's self and to expertise.

Public health and risk

The sociology of public health has been strongly influenced by Foucault's concepts, particularly his work on the body and governmentality. David Armstrong, whose work draws heavily on Foucault's earlier writings, emphasises the surveillance implications of public health interventions. In his seminal book, *Political Anatomy of the Body* (1983), he highlighted the political significance of a twentieth-century shift in the conception of the body, from a docile entity that could be used and transformed to a view of it as a subject and relative entity. The rise of new medical techniques, such as the survey, the controlled clinical trial, and epidemiology and specialisations (e.g. paediatrics, geriatrics, psychiatry) signalled a growing preoccupation with monitoring 'the social spaces between bodies' rather than the individual body. Like other writers, such as Sawicki, Armstrong emphasises the positive and productive power of the new forms of knowledge and techniques of surveillance and measurement. Such knowledge and techniques have allowed for the extension of 'normalisation', the process of measuring differences and specifying deviations from some idealised norm. In his later work, Armstrong drew on the work of Foucault and the anthropologist Mary Douglas to examine the 'shifts in the form and object of hygienic rules' operating in the regimes of public health, from the 'cordon sanitaire' of quarantine regulations to the monitored spaces of the 'new' public health (Armstrong, 1993). As Armstrong argued, each regime created spaces within which individual identity has been located.

The current emphasis on 'obesity' within populations exemplifies the preoccupation with body classification in modern societies highlighted by Foucault and others who draw on his ideas. Official measures of body mass (BMI) have been used universally, regardless of their cultural applicability (views on 'ideal' body size and shape vary considerably cross-culturally and through time), creating an 'obesity epidemic' requiring official intervention through efforts to physically modify bodies, change diets and increase levels of exercise (Petersen, 2007: 48–61). Measures such as BMI, and techniques for monitoring and controlling obesity – self-weighing (sometimes obsessively), the use of weight-loss treatments, including diets, exercise, liposuction, gastric banding and so on – construct the 'obese' subject who is called upon, as a 'responsible' citizen, to play a role in managing 'the problem' through engaging in practices of self-care and risk management. 'Excessive' weight and a failure to achieve a prescribed body size and shape are seen to signify an absence of control, poor decision making and social failure (Crawford, 1994). Many public health measures involve such normalisation and serve to change views on what constitutes a 'normal, healthy' body. The recent emergence of population-wide genetic databases – 'biobanks' – in many countries highlights this continuing effort to normalise the body and its health. Employing the techniques of genetic epidemiology, the purported aim of developing such collections is to ascertain the genetic and environmental contributions to disease, the underlying assumption being that there is some 'ideal', normal state of health and that, given enough data (read genetic information), new medicines can be developed that can be 'tailored' to individuals' genetic profile (so-called 'personalised medicines'), or that public health interventions can be devised to prevent illness in those who are deemed 'susceptible' in the future.

A growing body of sociological writings on public health and health promotion from the 1990s owes much to Foucault. Writers have drawn on Foucault's ideas and that of his followers (e.g. Castel,1991; Petersen and Lupton, 1996; Armstrong, 1993) to help make sense of the discourses and practices of the so-called new public health, such as those related to self-care, the healthy cities movement, community participation, healthy public policy and inter-sectoral collaboration. A number of new books on public health and health promotion appearing during the 1990s drew heavily on Foucault's concepts, particularly governmentality, regulation and 'technologies of the self'. These include Robin Bunton et al.'s *The Sociology of Health Promotion: Critical Analyses of Consumption, Lifestyle and Risk* (1995), Deborah Lupton's *The Imperative of Health: Public Health and the Regulated Body*

(1995), Alan Petersen and Deborah Lupton's *The New Public Health: Health and Self in the Age of Risk* (1996), and chapters within Alan Petersen and Robin Bunton's *Foucault, Health and Medicine* (1997). This body of work emerged in the context of the growing significance of neo-liberal rule in everyday life, involving a retreat of the welfare state, a growing emphasis on care of the self, and the rise of policies and practices (e.g. 'non-directive' counselling) that seek to enhance individual autonomy and 'freedom of choice'.

Foucault's concepts have proved useful in making sense of the field of public health and health promotion because they help reveal the exercise of power that underlies the numerous injunctions and practices that are presented as being for 'the public good' or 'the individual good'. Much public health is about educating the public on the dangers of undertaking certain 'risky' activities, or encouraging citizens to play a greater role in looking after their own health. These include limiting exposure to ultraviolet rays, reducing intake of alcohol and tobacco, eating 'healthily', engaging in 'safe sex' and so on. While these practices may appear to be self-evidently beneficial, in terms of advancing the health of individuals and society at large, as Foucauldian scholars point out, it is important to recognise that they always involve the exercise of power, being linked to broader governmental objectives. As noted, the Foucauldian concept of governmentality postulates an inextricable connection between 'practices of the self' and 'techniques of domination'. Thus, citizens are 'made up' in ways that accord with particular structures and configurations of power.

The concept of governmentality has proved valuable in the sociology of risk that grew significantly in the 1990s in the wake of the publication in English of Ulrich Beck's influential *The Risk Society* (1992). Beck, along with Giddens (e.g. 1991) and a number of other scholars of modernity, see risk as an aspect of 'reflexive modernisation', whereby modern societies seek to manage the environmental and social harms resulting from industrialisation. Foucauldians, on the other hand, view risk as an aspect of a particular mode of governance, namely neo-liberal governance. An early influential Foucauldian contribution in this regard is offered by Robert Castel (1991) in his article 'From dangerousness to risk', where he charts the development of new preventive strategies of social administration in a number of countries. As Castel argues, earlier modes of surveillance involving particular classes of subject (e.g. the carer and the cared for, and the professional and the client) increasingly are replaced by a combination of the 'factors of risk' measured by statistical correlations of diverse elements. Castel drew attention to the social costs of risk discourse, which entails a kind of 'witch hunt', a perpetual process of 'pulling up weeds', which constructs new risks, which constitutes novel targets for preventive intervention. From this Foucauldian perspective, risk is productive, in that it creates new classifications (e.g. the 'at risk' child, women 'at risk' of giving birth to a disabled child) and thus new fields for intervention and control. The concept of governmentality has been employed in the analysis of various risk-related phenomena in the field of health and more widely; e.g. mental illness, teenage pregnancy, post-menopausal diseases (e.g. Harding, 1997; Petersen, 1997; Petersen and Wilkinson, 2008).

Biological citizenship

The idea that people are 'made up' in particular ways through classifications reflects the Foucauldian notion that the human subject (generally known as 'the person', 'the individual' or 'human being') is a specific historical and social construction. This idea has been developed extensively by Ian Hacking, in his much-cited article, 'Making up people' (1986), and various books such as *The Taming of Chance* (1990), *The Social Construction of What?* (1999) and *Rewriting the Soul: Multiple Personality and the Science of Memory* (1995). Hacking proposed the term 'dynamic nominalism' to emphasise the dynamic relationship between the classifications and the self-conceptions, dispositions and actions of those who are so classified (Hacking, 1986). With the rapid growth of the 'new genetics' and other biosciences (e.g. neuroscience, stem cell science, nanoscience) in the 1990s and early 2000s, a number of social scientists have become interested in how the related new knowledge is shaping identity and experience (e.g. Petersen and Bunton, 2002; Bunton and Petersen, 2005; Rose, 1999). It has been noted that, increasingly, new identities and forms of sociability are evolving that involve an *active* relationship to the biosciences and biotechnologies.

An influential work in this regard is that by Adriana Petryna. In her book, *Life Exposed: Biological Citizens After Chernobyl* (2002), Petryna highlighted the significance of the forms of solidarity and activism based on biological criteria for victims of Chernobyl. In making their case for redress resulting from nuclear contamination, victims have needed to create a shared identity in order to stake their claims. The concept 'biological citizens' used by Petryna highlights the importance of biological criteria in citizens' self-conceptions and actions to draw attention to and improve their situation. The term 'biological citizenship', to express the resultant forms of citizen activism, has been developed further by Nicholas Rose and Carlos Novas (2005) to analyse the dynamics of patient activism, whereby patients develop an active relationship to biomedical knowledge, by developing online communities and using various media in their efforts to learn about and manage everyday life in relation to their condition. As this work emphasises, those who are ill employ a whole range of techniques of the self in their efforts to become well. Through their engagements with diverse information sources (e.g. 'direct-to-consumer' advertising), expert sources, other patients, lobbying and fundraising, patients develop an active relationship with science and related expertise. They thereby express and contribute to 'a political economy of hope' (Delvecchio Good *et al.*, 1990; Rose and Novas, 2005: 451–54). The concept of 'biological citizenship' proves useful in analysing the diverse discourse of 'healthy living', such as pertains to the HIV-affected individual and adherence to guidelines for healthy living. (On the utility of this concept, see Petersen *et al.* 2010, the special issue 'Healthy living and citizenship', in *Critical Public Health*.)

The practices of health and medicine

Foucault's work has been extensively employed in the analysis of the practices of health and medicine, including caring work (e.g. nursing), doctor–patient interactions and the 'medicalisation' of conditions, identities and behaviours. In his major contribution in this field of medical knowledge, *The Birth of the Clinic: An Archaeology of Medical Perception* (1975), Foucault described how modern medicine brought about a reorientation between the visible and the invisible, creating new classes of phenomena previously imperceptible and thus indescribable. What he referred to as the 'medical gaze' involved the reorganisation of space, in particular the hospital, the fabrication of the new identity of the patient, a new conception of the body (noted above) and new classifications of diseases and their signs and symptoms. The practices of dissection, for example, enabled physicians to understand the workings of the body in novel ways. In its modern history, anatomical instruction has played a central role in forging the identity of medicine – a fact that is becoming more evident with the emergence of new technologies and learning methods that do not involve dissection, such as the use of peer assessment, and the resulting resistance by some sections of the medical profession (Regan de Bere and Petersen, 2009). Foucault's concept of bio-power drew attention to the inescapably political character of biological knowledge, including related systems of classification, referred to earlier. Thus, the International Classifications of Diseases (ICD) and the Diagnostic and Statistical Manual of Mental Disorders (DSM), which are formal biomedical classifications of morbidity and mortality and mental disorders, respectively, can be seen as technologies of the medical gaze, generating new, previously medically unrecognised conditions subject to diagnosis and treatments according to supposedly objective criteria. These classificatory schemes are periodically revised and applied internationally, emphasising the ways in which biomedicine may 'colonise' conditions, identities and behaviours (and territories) over time.

Foucauldian scholarship offers a critical perspective on practices of care, showing that purportedly benevolent policies, such as 'patient-centred' medicine, and the practice of 'getting to know' the patient as an 'individual' or 'whole person' in nursing involve the subtle exercise of power. Rather than democratising the unequal relationship between patients and carers, such policies may in fact serve to draw patients into processes of their own surveillance and control (e.g. May, 1992: 485–86). This involves what Foucault describes as 'pastoral power', which appears benevolent – guiding people towards happiness – but can be seen to serve as a mechanism of control. In his *The Social Meaning of Surgery* (1992), Nicholas Fox examined how surgical power operates through the techniques at the surgeon's command. In his exploration of the post-operative ward round, for example, Fox shows how surgeon–patient interactions allow surgeons to manage the discourse on healing to maintain their power and authority. Patients are offered few opportunities to intervene or introduce their own agenda for interaction (Fox, 1992: 77–93; see also Fox, 1993).

Foucault's ideas have proved highly insightful for those who have sought to develop new ways of understanding the operations and implications of biomedical power, including the phenomenon of medicalisation that has long been of interest to sociologists; e.g. Zola (1972), Conrad and Schneider (1992). A growing number of scholars have recognised the limitations and implications of modernist theoretical perspectives for understanding the power relations of biomedicine. Biomedical perspectives involve reductionism – a tendency to see complex problems, involving many facets (socio-cultural, psycho-social and biophysical; e.g. mental illness), as reducible to biophysical malfunction and as consequently treatable through interventions such as drugs and surgery. However, sociology as the study of 'society' may itself be reductive, in overemphasising socio-cultural constraints. As Foucauldian scholars have pointed out, power operates not so much through overt control (repression) (e.g. doctor–patient interactions), but through its particular 'productive' capacity, which leads to problems being defined and dealt with in a limited number of ways. Writers working in fields such as disability studies have used a number of Foucauldian concepts in their efforts to overcome the limitations of biomedicine's (and sociology's) reductionism and underlying dualistic conceptions, such as nature–culture, mind–body, structure–agency, natural–unnatural, and normal–abnormal.

The discourses of disability

In recent years, scholars have drawn on Foucault's ideas to challenge the discourses of disability, including notions of the natural and the ethical and the idea of liberation (Tremain, 2005: 2). For example, the concepts of 'bio-politics' and 'bio-power', introduced in Volume One of *The History of Sexuality* (1976), have been usefully applied in this field to show how classifications (e.g. 'the deaf person', 'the mentally defective person') and associated practices and procedures (e.g. forms of treatment, care and support) serve to construct 'normal' and 'abnormal' bodies and mental abilities and operate as mechanisms of governance. The genealogical method has proved insightful in revealing how phenomena such as personality disorders and child mental health are historically and socially constructed (e.g. McCallum, 1997; Tyler, 1997). Recent studies, implicitly or explicitly drawing on Foucault's ideas, have questioned the dualistic thinking underlying theoretical approaches to disability and responses to associated discrimination. As Tom Shakespeare (2006), a prominent UK disability scholar, argues, disability studies has been dominated by the social model of disability, which has been a reaction against the medical model. This model makes a distinction between 'impairment' (the objectively defined physical or mental condition) and 'disability', which is a social creation. (On this distinction, also see Hughes, 2005.) This model, however, overlooks the fact that disability is the outcome of the complex interaction between individual and structural factors. Eliminating 'social barriers' does not resolve all the problems encountered by disabled people, whose experience is likely to be profoundly shaped by the impairment, the costs associated with work, welfare and poverty, and the natural effects of the ageing process (Shakespeare, 2006: 67). Foucauldian-inspired scholarship in the disability studies field has explored how disabled bodies and identities are constructed and regulated through, for example, regimes of body maintenance, therapeutic control, techniques of the confession and practices of (self-) care (e.g. Campbell, 2009; Sullivan, 2005; Yates, 2005). Policy responses to disability that seem enlightened and liberating, such as policies of de-institutionalisation and 'supported living', it has been suggested, may represent the dispersal and intensification of power (see, e.g. Drinkwater, 2005). Foucauldian-inspired work of this kind is valuable in showing that the classifications of disability are historically contingent and may serve as tools of governance.

Limitations of Foucault's work and related scholarship

While Foucault's work has proved invaluable in social studies of health and healthcare, it has some 'blindspots' that one should not overlook. Foucault's ideas are highly alluring – one could say 'sexy' – and over the last two decades a substantial field of scholarship has grown up around his work that is often difficult for 'outsiders' to infiltrate. One problem relates to the use of a specialised language. Terms like 'governmentality', 'technologies of self' and 'disciplinary' are used liberally by many scholars influenced by Foucault, which sometimes leads to confusion in discussion. Some of Foucault's terms were poorly defined and do not translate easily into English. A number of his concepts, such as 'resistance', were left under-theorised and one has to make interpretations as to their meaning from scattered writings and interviews. This difficulty posed by language use is not trivial and it is not limited to Foucauldian scholarship; however, it seems particularly acute in this field. Language is of crucial significance when scholars seek to engage with policymakers and other influential decision makers in order to shape policy agendas. There is much in Foucault's work that can usefully inform thinking about policies impacting on health and healthcare, including issues of risk management and governance. However, scholarship will fail to have policy significance if writers are unable to clearly communicate their ideas with those outside their field.

A major limitation of Foucault's work and that of many of his followers is the tendency to provide inadequate attention to individual and group agency, contestation and counter-discourse. The focus on 'discourse' and 'governance' and 'top-down' rule can lead to an emphasis on domination and to overlook the failures of governance and 'bottom-up' processes of subversion and resistance. As a number of writers have argued, this bias in much Foucauldian scholarship has left writers open to the charge of reinforcing state-centred views of government (e.g. Garland, 1997; O'Malley, et al., 1997; Stenson, 1998). As Garland argues, it is not meaningful to analyse abstract rationalities without investigating how they function in practice (1997: 200). Foucauldian scholarship would benefit from connecting with critical theory, in order to make it politically relevant. While there has been an understandable rejection of grand theory, such as that associated with Marxism, drawing on other schools of thought can enrich Foucauldian scholarship by providing deeper, more nuanced analyses of socio-political processes.

In particular, Foucauldian scholarship has been inattentive to the workings of political economy and to the significance of gender, ethnicity and socio-economic status or class in shaping experience. A strong emphasis on the workings of governance in relation to health and medical practices, such as those associated with 'healthy living' (Petersen *et al.*, 2010), has led scholars to overlook the substantial role played by powerful industry interests, including diverse media, in shaping discourses of health, illness and the body. An understanding of political economy is not incompatible with governmentality scholarship, which has been strongly concerned with the 'rationalities' of neo-liberal rule. Neo-liberalism is a manifestation of late, free-market capitalism, and we need to better understand how the particular forms of governance associated with contemporary health and medicine and healthcare reflect and are shaped by the dynamics of global politico-economy. Earlier contributions in the political economy of health (e.g. Doyal and Pennell, 1979) could be complemented and updated by a nuanced understanding of the dynamics of neo-liberal rule. This would be useful in analysing global developments such as 'direct-to-consumer' advertising of medical goods and services, which challenge state-centred conceptions of power and regulation and are premised upon particular constructions of the human subject and subjectivity.

All theories and concepts should be open to modification and change. Indeed, one would expect this to happen as society itself changes. Theories and thinkers are subject to cycles of fashion, and in sociology one can trace shifts in theoretical interest over time, reflecting wider trends in the economy, culture, and politics and policy. Interest in Marxism, phenomenology, symbolic interactionism and different schools of feminism has risen and fallen and been replaced by postmodernism, poststructuralism and postcolonial theory as reflection upon the inadequacies of earlier theories has become apparent. French theorists such as Baudrillard, Deleuze, Bourdieu and Foucault became fashionsionable in the late 1980s and 1990s, much like Marx, Fridan and Goffman were fashionable in the 1960s and 1970s. Despite the passing of almost 30 years since his death, Foucault continues to inspire since he left such a rich legacy of ideas pertaining to many areas of social life. While the Foucault effect has been profound, we should guard against dogmatism and the myth that there can be one, all-encompassing theory to explain the complexity of modern life. We should use Foucault's work as he intended – as a *toolbox of ideas*, to inspire us and help us reflect upon contemporary society. I like the toolbox metaphor, which I keep in mind as go about my own research. I continue to be inspired by Foucault, although I do not use his concepts as self-consciously as I did when I was first introduced to his writings many years ago. I hope you, too, will find his ideas insightful and put them to work in novel ways to help make sense of health and healthcare, which directly or indirectly affect everyone.

Further useful reading

Weblink

michel-foucault.com: http://www.michel-foucault.com/info/about.html

References

Armstrong, D. (1983) *Political Anatomy of the Body: Medical Knowledge in Britain in the Twentieth Century*. Cambridge University Press: Cambridge.

——(1993) 'Public health spaces and the fabrication of identity', *Sociology*, 27, 3: 39–401.
Barrett, M. (1991) *The Politics of Truth: From Marx to Foucault*. Polity Press: Cambridge.
Beck, U. (1992) *The Risk Society: Towards a New Modernity*. Sage: London.
Bunton, R. and Petersen, A. (eds) (2005) *Genetic Governance: Health, Risk and Ethics in the Biotech Era*. Routledge: London.
Bunton, R., Nettleton, S. and Burrows, R. (1995) *The Sociology of Health Promotion: Critical Analyses of Consumption, Lifestyle and Risk*. Routledge: London.
Campbell, F. K. (2009) *Contours of Ableism: The Production of Disability and Ableness*. Palgrave Macmillan: Houndmills.
Castel, R. (1991) 'From dangerousness to risk', in G. Burchell, C. Gordon and N. Rose (eds.) *The Foucault Effect: Studies in Governmentality*. Harvester Wheatsheaf: Hemel Hempstead.
Conrad, P. and Schneider, J. W. (1992) *Deviance and Medicalization: From Badness to Sickness*, expanded edition. Temple University Press: Philadelphia, PA.
Corea, G. (1985) *The Mother Machine: Reproductive Technologies From Artificial Insemination to Artificial Wombs*. Harper and Row: New York.
Crawford, R. (1994) 'The boundaries of the self and the unhealthy other: reflections on health, culture and AIDS', *Social Science and Medicine*, 38, 10: 1347–65.
Dean, M. (1999) *Governmentality: Power and Rule in Modern Society*. Sage: New York.
Delvecchio Good, M-J., Good, B.J., Schaffer, C. and Lind, S. E. (1990) 'American oncology and the discourse on hope', *Culture, Medicine and Psychiatry*, 14: 59–79.
Doyal, L. and Pennell, L. (1979) *The Political Economy of Health*. Pluto Press: London.
Drinkwater, C. (2005) 'Supported living and the production of individuals', in S. Tremain (ed.) *Foucault and the Government of Disability*. The University of Michigan Press: Michigan.
Flax, J. (1990) *Thinking Fragments; Psychoanalysis, Feminism, and Postmodernism in the Contemporary West*. University of California Press: Berkeley.
Foucault, M. (1975) *The Birth of the Clinic: An Archaeology of Medical Perception*. Vintage Books: New York.
——(1977) *Discipline and Punish: The Birth of the Prison*. Penguin: Harmondsworth.
——(1980) *The History of Sexuality*. Vol. One. *An Introduction*. Vintage Books: New York.
——(1985) *The Use of Pleasure*, trans. R. Hurley. Penguin: Harmondsworth.
——(1986) *The Care of the Self*, trans. R. Hurley. Penguin: Harmondsworth.
Fox, N. (1992) *The Social Meaning of Surgery*. Open University Press: Buckingham.
——(1993) 'Discourse, organisation, and the surgical ward round', *Sociology of Health and Illness*, 15, 1: 16–42.
Garland, D. (1997) 'Governmentality and the problem of crime: Foucault, criminology, sociology', *Theoretical Criminology*, 1, 2: 173–214.
Giddens, A. (1991) *Modernity and Self-Identity: Self and Society in the Late Modern Age*. Polity: Cambridge.
Hacking, I. (1986) 'Making up people', in T. C. Heller, M. Sosna and D. E. Wellberg (eds) *Reconstructing Individualism: Autonomy, Individuality and the Self in Western Thought*. Stanford University Press: Standford, CA.
——(1990) *The Taming of Chance*. Cambridge: Cambridge University Press.
——(1995) *Rewriting the Soul: Multiple Personality and the Sciences of Memory*. Princeton University Press: Princeton, NJ.
——(1999) *The Social Construction of What?* Cambridge, MA: Haward University Press.
Harding, J. (1997) 'Bodies at risk: sex, surveillance and hormone replacement therapy', in A. Petersen and R. Bunton (eds) *Foucault, Health and Medicine*. Routledge: London.
Hughes, B. (2005) 'What can a Foucauldian analysis contribute to disability theory?', in S. Tremain (ed.) *Foucault and the Government of Disability*. The University of Michigan Press: Michigan.

Lupton, D. (1995) *The Imperative of Health: Public Health and the Regulated Body*. Sage: London.
May, C. (1992) 'Nursing work, nurses' knowledge, and the subjectification of the patient', *Sociology of Health and Illness*, 14, 4: 472–87.
McCallum, D. (1997) 'Mental health, criminality and the human sciences', in A. Petersen and R. Bunton (eds) *Foucault, Health and Medicine*. Routledge: London and New York.
Murtagh, M. (2003) 'Feminist ethics and menopause: autonomy and decision-making in primary medical care', *Social Science & Medicine* 56, 8: 1643–1652.
Petersen, A. (1997) 'Risk, governance and the new public health', in A. Petersen and R. Bunton (eds) *Foucault, Health and Medicine*. Routledge: London.
——(2007) *The Body in Question: A Socio-Cultural Approach*. Routledge: London.
Petersen, A. and Bunton, R. (2002) *The New Genetics and the Public's Health*. Routledge: London.
——(eds) (1997) *Foucault, Health and Medicine*. Routledge: London.
Petersen, A. and Lupton, D. (1996) *The New Public Health: Health and Self in the Age of Risk*. Allen and Unwin: North Sydney, and Sage: London.
Petersen, A. and Wilkinson, I. (eds) (2008) *Health, Risk and Vulnerability*. Routledge: London.
Petersen, A., Davis, M., Fraser, S. and Lindsay, J. (2010) 'Healthy living and citizenship: an overview', *Critical Public Health*, 20, 4: 1–10.
Petryna, A. (2002) *Life Exposed: Biological Citizens After Chernobyl*. Princeton University Press: Princeton, NJ.
Regan de Bere, S. and Petersen, A. (2009) 'Crisis or renaissance? A sociology of anatomy in UK medical education', C. Brosman and B. Turner (eds) *Handbook of the Sociology of Medical Education*. Routledge: London.
Robertson, M. (1992) *Starving in the Silences: An Exploration of Anorexia Nervosa*. Allen Biological citizenship', in A. Ong and S. J. Collier (eds) *Global Assemblages: Technology, Politics, and Ethics As Anthropological Problems*. Blackwell Publishing: Malden, MA.
Rowse, T. (1998) *White Flour, White Power; From Rations to Citizenship in Central Australia*. Cambridge University Press: Cambridge.
Sawicki, J. (1991) *Disciplining Foucault: Feminism, Power and the Body*. Routledge: New York.
Seear, K. (2009) 'The etiquette of endometriosis: Stigmatisation, menstrual concealment and the diagnostic delay', Social Science 27.
Shakespeare, T. (2006) *Disability Rights and Wrongs*. Routledge: London.
Stenson, J. (1998) Beyond histories of the present. *Economy and Society*, 27, 4: 333–352.
Sullivan, M. (2005) 'Subjected bodies: paraplegia, rehabilitation and the politics of movement', in S. Tremain (ed.) *Foucault and the Government of Disability*. The University of Michigan Press: Michigan.
Tremain, S. (ed.) (2005) *Foucault and the Government of Disability*. The University of Michigan Press: Michigan.
Tyler, D. (1997) 'At risk of maladjustment: the problem of child mental health', in A. Petersen and R. Bunton (eds) *Foucault, Health and Medicine*. Routledge: London.
Yates, S. (2005) 'Truth, power and ethics in care services for people with learning difficulties', in S. Tremain (ed.) *Foucault and the Government of Disability*. The University of Michigan Press: Michigan.
Zola, I. (1972) 'Medicine as an institution of social control', *The Sociological Review*, 20, 4: 487–504.

2 Consuming bodies: Zygmunt Bauman on the difference between fitness and health

Paul Higgs

This chapter is concerned with examining the contribution of the work of Zygmunt Bauman to the understanding of health and embodiment in contemporary societies. Of necessity this will be a prismatic reading of a writer whose capacity to produce often more than one book a year can overwhelm anyone trying to get a grip on his overall thought. Certainly an assessment of the variety of manifestations of 'liquid modernity' put forward in Bauman's work, including its relationship to post-modernism, is outside the scope of what is presented here. Instead what I propose to do is to examine the utility of Bauman's use of the idea of 'fitness' in work that has a considerable bearing on both medical sociology and the sociology of the body. The potential insights offered by his understanding of the notion of fitness has played an important role in elaborating the way that consumer society has transformed the nature of what health is and how it functions in a world where many of our normative assumptions about life have been challenged by changes that ultimately lead to the emergence of a liquid modernity. By outlining this particular dimension of how individuals have to confront embodiment in the face of insatiable demands for perfection, a new point of departure can be created for the sociology of health and illness.

Freedom and consumption

However, before we go into a deeper examination of the idea of fitness and how it re-orientates our ideas of health, we need to first briefly situate the development of Bauman's thought and how it has come to represent part of a new canon of sociological thought (Outhwaite 2009). While having published extensively on a whole number of topics since the 1960s, a large part of his work up until the 1990s was concerned with the role of rationality in the development of what we have come to know as modernity. Consequently one of Bauman's most praised works, *Modernity and the Holocaust* (Bauman 1989), concerned itself with the ways in which these processes, connected with the drive to create order in modern life, led in the case of Germany to the horrors of the Holocaust. Since the 1990s Bauman's main interest, however, has been the relationship between the post-modernisation of society and the growth of consumerism. These two periods are not as disconnected as they might seem at first sight given that a common concern has been the marginalisation of the other, whether organised around the categories of ethnic origins or failed consumers. Consequently this concern for the negative effects on groups of individuals, resulting from which might otherwise be seen as neutral processes, has been a hallmark of Bauman's work, and helps situate his thinking against the more celebrated approaches adopted by other writers dealing with similar material, such as Anthony Giddens and Jean Baudrillard (Blackshaw, 2005; Smith, 1999). In a similar fashion to these writers Bauman does see a dramatic change in the organising principles of late twentieth and early twenty-first century Western societies. Not only have many of the stable institutions of the modernist nation-state been transformed from within through processes such as deindustrialisation, women's employment, reconfiguration of domestic relationships and social mobility, but so also has the key defining relationship of employment. Bauman sees this transformation as being one from a 'society of producers' to a 'society of consumers' (Bauman, 1995). Again this might be seen as both trite and lacking in theoretical insight, but unlike Baudrillard for example this view is not mainly about its epistemological consequences but rather needs to be viewed in terms of its ontological implications. These ontological implications are mainly to be found in how consumption operates and in what ways individuals respond to the interpellations of consumer society. A large factor in this is the way in which consumption appears to be based on the creation and maintenance of anxieties that are created not only through the operation of the market but as a consequence of the valorisation of choice.

The transformation of modern societies from ones built around producers and the needs of production to ones centred on consumers and consumption is a development that Bauman has addressed in a number of works, as he has wrestled with the implications of how individuals negotiate a world that has not developed along the lines that his previously self-identified position as a Marxist expected (Smith, 1999). This is particularly true in relation to those areas of social structure such as social class that were seen as foundational to modernity and capitalism. In his work on *Freedom* (Bauman, 1988) Bauman made the argument that the real distinction in modern society was to be found in whether individuals had the capacity to make choices in a consumer market or not. In recent years this capability had become more important as in the past the provision of public goods by the state was seen to be a valid form of consumption, constituting part of the 'social wage' provided to the working class as compensation for the inequalities generated in market societies; in the contemporary world this provision now marked out individuals as 'failed consumers' whose consumption was deemed invalid. According to Bauman, to be a recipient of public services or benefits rather than consumer products indicated to others a fundamental lack of capacity. This argument did not alter with regard to the nature of these services or benefits, nor whether they were either the same or better than those provided by the market. Instead what mattered was that they could not be seen to be the outcome of choice or agency. This 'flaw' in 'socialised' consumption has been projected onto social housing and onto the public provision of health services as well as pensions. In part it is amplified by the mass media who at all levels have an interest in encouraging consumer markets, but it also has its echoes in the lives of many users of public services who have had to accept the imposition of the decisions of public service bureaucracies on mundane issues, such as the colour of front doors as well as more important decisions regarding treatment options and restrictions in health and social care.

Developing this theme further, Bauman has argued in his *Work, consumerism and the new poor* (Bauman, 1998a) that the emergence of an extensive consumer society not only gives rise to the idea that those who most rely on public support are to some degree lesser citizens because of their existence as failed consumers, but that as the whole social world has re-orientated itself around consumption they in fact, paradoxically, become the only section of society to be viewed in terms of their capacity to work. This paradox has its origins in a transformation of one of the fundamental axioms of the 'society of producers', namely the work ethic. Here the assumption is that there is a connection between wealth and work, with higher and more distinctive levels of consumption being an outcome of the more rewarding employment enjoyed by those in higher status occupations. In the society of consumers this assumption no longer necessarily holds. Consumption is an increasing end in itself to be enjoyed as a form of display for others to engage with. How people earn the money to pay for this consumption or indeed whether they are 'worth' the incomes that sustain the most expensive parts of this world is no longer a key part of the moral economy of most people's lives, rather this is seen as a part of the fundamental differentiation of the world, which may be seen as fair or unfair but with no fundamental connection to an ordered system of occupations. However, this is not true for those occupying postitions outside of employment and who have to apply or be dependent upon public or state funds. For them their status as welfare recipients makes them both 'failed consumers' and people whose lives need to be situated against the need to find work. In contemporary society it is those who need to be provided with resources to consume who find that they need to demonstrate a 'work ethic'; welfare policy is now organised around the theme of labour market activation, and proposed reforms to entitlements now routinely see the issues as ones of motivating individuals into the habits of working, whether or not this may be suitable or indeed possible.

From the society of producers to the society of consumers

The shift from the society of producers to the society of consumers also bears down on the issues of health and illness. Bauman in his work on the Holocaust is very aware of how the imagery of disease and infection can be used to justify policies that not only exclude others but which can also lead to their elimination or potential extermination. This capacity that emerges as an aspect of the rationalising process of modernity connects with the role of the modern nation-state as an entity to organise and respond to the problems emerging from industrialisation and urbanisation. Part of this response was the need to create policies for the mass of the population, which brought to bear technical solutions in order to maximise the potential benefits as well as minimise anticipated risks. In this way we can see the emergence not only of modern healthcare systems, with their divisions between hospitals and general practice, but also the creation of public and enviromental health as particular specialities. These institutions were created in addition to the development of universal education and welfare by the nation-state. Important for Bauman is the recognition that while many of these institutions still continue to the present, the functions that they currently carry out are transformed by the shift towards the society of consumers. In particular the focus has shifted from the collective to the individual. In a memorable image Bauman describes how

> The huge State-wide garden has been split into innumerable small allotments. What used to be done in a condensed and concentrated fashion, through universal laws instilled thanks to the state's normative fervour and guarded by the state police, is now done in an uncoordinated way by commercial companies, quasi-tribal groups, or the individuals themselves. We are, as before, striving for rationality, but this is now a micro-rationality (or rather micro-rationalities – as a rule acting at cross purposes, clashing with each other, refusing to merge or so much as compromise), which cannot but which 'produce irrationality at the level of the whole'.
>
> (Bauman, 1995: 173–74)

Health fits into this schema by Bauman situating its historical development within the emergence and transformation of modernity. For Bauman in the era of the society of producers the idea of the standardised body is required by both industry and the military. The standardised body was an outcome of the processes of modernisation, which wished to minimise the 'uncertainty' that dominated the pre-modern world by means of the creation of a rationalised order. 'Order' was now to be the prime motivation in directing public actions, whether this was in the context of the manufacture of goods or whether it was in the conduct of warfare. Drawing on Foucault's use of Jeremy Bentham's concept of the Panopticon, Bauman sees the transformation of the modern world as being one in which the surveillance of the population's everyday activities, whether at work, home or school, becomes a day-to-day reality of modernist rationality, leaving only as he puts it 'the small stretches at the beginning and the end – where whatever uncertainty might be experienced was not seen as a "social problem"' (Bauman, 1995: 109).

Bauman sees the 'regimentation' of society under the society of producers as intimately connected to the emergence of panics about the 'physical deterioration' and condition of bodies of the working classes by both the state and by the emerging institutions of modern society. He points out that the real concern that underlay this awareness was less a common humanitarian impulse and more a concern with the maintenance of social order and the prevention of a return of the 'problem of vagrancy'. Consequently in terms that have contemporary resonance, the lack of health displayed by the unemployed and the would-be soldiers did not just reflect personal problems of ill health, but indicated a potential national loss that needed to be overcome by surveillance, measurement and a re-orientation towards tasks that would ultimately reintegrate such outlying groups into their primary purpose as constituting potential workers or soldiers. However, as Bauman points out, neither labouring nor being a soldier are much in need today, or not in the numbers they once were. The 'regime of regimentation' as he terms it is also falling out of favour as is the 'uniformity of behaviour' and the underpinning social desire to 'conform'. Instead the reproduction of the conditions of social life are now to a large extent privatised – removed from 'the realm of state politics and, indeed, of public decision-making' (Bauman, 1995: 113). It is to the individual that decisions about self-formation are left. Whereas in the past, according to Bauman, the fear of uncertainty needed the Bentham-inspired Panopticon to ensure cooperation and the avoidance of deviation, and counter to the Foucault of *Discipline and Punish* (Foucault, 1977) contemporary society deals with the same fears through the processes of what he calls 'privatisation'.

> Processes are now by and large *de-institutionalized*, building up from the grass-roots level out of the individual DIY efforts at self-formation.
> (Bauman, 1995: 113)

A number of consequences flow from this shift. Not only is there a move from what are described as 'because ofs' to 'in order tos' in the nature of individuals' lives, but also the fear of inadequacy replaces the idea of deviation. Inadequacy also changes from being a 'clear cut and solid standard' to one that is much more elusive. Bauman explains this new inadequacy in the following terms:

> ... [it is] the sense of failing to acquire the shape and form one wished to acquire, whatever that form might have been; failing to stay on the move but also failing to stop at the spot of one's choice, to stay flexible and ready to assume shapes at will, to be simultaneously pliable clay and accomplished sculptor.
> (Bauman, 1995: 113)

Moreover, conformity is replaced by an overarching and determining 'meta-effort', which is seen as the necessary effort to stay fit in order to be able to demonstrate that the individual is making efforts not to get stuck in any one location for too long. Bauman is aware that there seems to be an elective affinity between this new state of affairs and consumer capitalism, with the market both feeding on the fears of insecurity and providing responses for them. Consequently, while what Bauman now describes as the 'regime of self-formation' seems to intensify the anxieties of uncertainty that the 'regime of surveillance' sought to control, it does so by offering a seeming freedom from responsibility. Choices are not outlived by their outcomes and these in turn do not necessarily 'prejudice episodes still to come' (1995: 114). Bauman sums it up in the following juxtaposition:

> Instead of the enforced, imposed irresponsibility of the prisoner (which weighs down heavily as deprivation and slavery), the irresponsibility of a

butterfly (which is worn lightly and joyously as gift and freedom). Light is where darkness once was; passage into new dependence feels like liberation, like 'getting out'.

(Bauman, 1995: 114)

It is not therefore surprising that Bauman links this transformation with the move from individuals being defined as 'goods-purveyors' to being seen as 'sensation gatherers'. The change reflects different articulating premises, with the former being collective and the latter being privatised. It is therefore relatively simple to see how the focus on heath and on the body begins to change. Health under the regime of surveillance was articulated around enabling the producer's or soldier's body. The capacity 'to respond to stimuli promptly and with the required vigour' amounted to 'health' while 'illness' was the obverse of this (1995: 115). Health was therefore seen in terms of various inputs and outputs maximised for optimal functioning. As an example of this Bauman points out that the first 'minimum standard of living' calculated by Seebohm Rowntree at the beginning of the twentieth century, which only included items of notional nutritional value and excluded tea because this was perceived to be a luxury item providing no sustenance and could therefore be accordingly be dispensed with. Under the regime of sensation gathering, bodies are seen first and foremost as 'consuming' bodies and their ontology is first and foremost the construction of the capacity to consume.

Fitness and health

By identifying the move to a society of consumers and the role played by consumer bodies we see the emergence of the important role that fitness starts to play in Bauman's thinking. Again quoting Bauman:

> The postmodern body is first and foremost a receiver of *sensations*, it imbibes and digests *experiences*; the capacity of being stimulated renders it an instrument of *pleasure*. That capacity is called fitness; obversely the 'state of unfitness' stands for langour, apathy, listlessness, dejection, a lackadaisical response to stimuli; for a shrinking or just 'below average' capacity for, and an interest in, new sensations and experiences.
>
> (Bauman, 1995: 116)

He writes that a 'fit' body is one that is tuned to pleasure. However, because the depth or intensity of pleasure cannot be measured, the notions of 'normality' and 'abnormality' created by modern medicine in order to put some order on the world start to become problematic. Unlike the recordability of 'normal temperature', the subjective experience of sensation is always open to the doubt that it has not matched up to what others experience. Bauman uses the telling metaphor of the fly in the ointment by pointing out that in every ointment of achievement 'there is a fly of suspicion that the actually felt experience was but a pale shadow of what the "real" experience could be (and if it *could*, it *should*)' (1995: 117). The importance of this is that not only is 'normality' undermined but that all sensations are subject to what he calls a 'sliding scale of pleasure', which views all experiences as aspects of 'malfunction' and in doing so creates the possibility for endless dissatisfaction.

For Bauman, the process of creating the 'truly fit' body is transfixed by unending anxiety caused by continuous disappointments and leading to feelings of perpetual inadequacy. In addition, he argues, the very individualisation of a consumer society cuts off the possibility of a social or political response that in the past was one of the ways of dealing with this unease. In particular, given that all problems are ultimately 'self-inflicted mishaps', there are no collective solutions or indeed any realistic forms of social redress. As he puts it: 'the drilling of the producer/soldier body unites: the self drill of the sensations-gatherer body divides and separates' (1995: 118). Furthermore Bauman points out that the body is now uncontested 'private property' and it is therefore up to the owner to cultivate it as well as to accept the blame for when things go wrong.

In *Life in Fragments* (Bauman, 1995), where Bauman first introduced the idea of fitness into his account of the changing world, the notion is used as a way of extending his concern with living in a fragmenting world. In another of his powerful images he argues that the 'modern' ideal of the body was one conceived along the lines of Renaissance notions of harmony, whereby all tensions and conflicts were ultimately removed and where there was no further possible improvement. In contrast, contemporary ideals of fitness adhere to a Gothic interpretation of the body so that it is 'composed of excesses alone and held together solely through finely balancing the tensions that tear it apart' (Bauman, 1995: 121). Bauman therefore asserts that as a result the individual owner of the contemporary body is now constantly in a state of siege balancing the tensions in a permanent process of dealing with disappointment.

This theme is continued in *Liquid Life* (Bauman, 2005), where Bauman locates the idea of fitness within the more developed paradigm he now terms 'Liquid Modernity'; in a similar vein to both Giddens and Beck he describes a modernity that is not only not solid but which has difficulties in creating institutions that can indeed solidify (Bauman, 2000). The fragmentation that this causes in individuals' lives is similar to that identified in his earlier work, with its focus on the individualisation of constant insecurity. Developing the connections between health and fitness and the role of the uncertainty provoked by consumer society, Bauman writes:

> 'Fitness' is to a consumer in the society of consumers what 'health' was to the society of producers. It is a certificate of 'being in', of belonging, of inclusion, of the right of residence. 'Fitness' knows no upper limit; it is, in fact, defined by the absence of limit … However fit your body is – *you could make it fitter*. However fit it may be at the moment, there is always a vexing helping of 'unfitness' mixed in, coming to light or guessed at whenever you compare what you have experienced with the pleasures suggested by the rumours and

sights of other people's joys which you have failed to experience thus far and can only imagine and dream of living through yourself. In the search for fitness, unlike in the case of health, there is no point at which you can say: now that I have reached it I may as well stop and hold onto and enjoy what I have. There is no 'norm' of fitness you can aim at and eventually attain.

(Bauman 2005: 93)

This passage points to a very important point being made by Bauman in his re-articulation of the relationship between health and fitness because it is pointing out that fitness is not an extension of health in the way that it is often used but rather a transcendence of it. The debates around what constituted health and what constituted illness, which have been a standard part of the sociology of health and illness as well as public health, have concentrated on whether the absence of disease is a sufficient condition for the existence of health or whether a more positive definition of human flourishing should be provided. These debates become hopelessly caught up in the previous social relationships of the standardised body typified by the society of producers. Bauman's reconfiguration points to a new relationship between illness, health and fitness, one that challenges the notions of 'normal' and 'abnormal' in terms of what health might be by introducing the unrealisable demands of fitness into the equation (Jones and Higgs, 2010). The impact of fitness on health does not stop here, however, the requirements necessary for the successful pursuit of fitness are equally uncertain. Again to quote Bauman:

Since the ideal of fitness offers only vague and uncertain rule-of-thumb instructions as to what is to be done and what is to be avoided, and since one can never be sure that the instructions won't change or even be revoked before you've managed to implement them in full, to struggle for fitness means never to rest; at any rate, never to *feel you can* rest with a clear conscience and without apprehension.

(Bauman, 2005: 94)

If the boundary between health and fitness has become confused by the random compulsiveness of the desire for fitness then it is equally true that the same process is going on in terms of definitions of illness, which under the previous regime were perceived to be more simple to understand, even if, on occasion, they reflected the interests of powerful groups or dominant discourses. The processes of medicalisation (Conrad and Potter, 2000) that have been extensively researched have demonstrated not only the presence of Illich's concepts of social and cultural iatrogenesis but also the transformation of 'underperformance' into medical problems and responses (Marshall and Katz, 2002). Medicalisation could be seen as another aspect of the impact of the shift to a society of consumers and the importance of the ideal of fitness. What constitutes illness and how it is dealt with now operate much more in the context of uncertainty and insecurity than they have done in the past, where Parsons' sick role held sway. Bauman understands this in terms of the increased significance of the somatic in the contemporary world. As he points out:

> The surface and the apertures of the body, all the vulnerable points in the boundary/interface that separates/links the body from/to the outside world, are therefore bound to become sites of ineradicable ambivalence.
> (Bauman, 2005: 95)

This ineradicable ambivalence allows the body to be a site of unknowable dangers that not only threaten but which cannot be prevented no matter how vigilant the individual is. Moreover, as the techniques of Armstrong's 'surveillance medicine' (Armstrong, 1995) become more and more the template of the 'imperative of health' (Lupton 1995), fear of the risks associated with modern life become more and more the underlying nature of illness, not yet revealed but present. Bauman cites the rise of our concern with 'fat', which he sees as encapsulating many of the issues reconstituting health:

> Fat has become a major war-cry and the *casus belli* in the 'culture war for the new century' ... The elevation of the 'fat issue' follows closely, and predictably, on the promotion of the consumer's body to the central target of marketing, and of the care of the body to the main selling point of consumer commodities.
> (Bauman, 2005: 98)

Body fat therefore represents a 'nightmare come true' and draws parallels, according to Bauman, with terrorism in that once ingested it takes control of the body and therefore needs to be resisted. The imagery may be overly dramatic but it does draw attention to what now gets seen as representing threats to health and the capacity to demonstrate fitness. The role of hydrogenated, saturated and unsaturated fats are all placed in a public debate as choices that have to be made alongside the informed choices that will lead you to lose weight and maintain the 'right' kind of metabolism. The consequences of not making the right kind of choices not only mean that you will put on weight but that also you are once again a flawed consumer. The 'illness' of being 'fat' is not just contained in the risk factors associated with it but also in being considered *homo sacer* (a person excepted from human as well as divine law) and considered an alien within the consumer society.

> The new and fast growing category of *homini sacri* specific to the liquid modern society of consumers is composed, as might be expected, of 'flawed' or failed consumers. Unlike indolent people in the society of producers, humans failed by the current standards of *bios* are not 'medical cases', candidates for treatment and rehabilitation, temporarily unfortunate but bound to be reassimilated sooner or later and readmitted to the community. They are truly and fully useless – redundant, supernumesary leftovers of a society

reconstituting itself as a society of consumers ... and so the 'community' would be so much better off were they to disappear ...

(Bauman, 2005: 100)

Although this might not be the fate of all conditions seen as illnesses, the cultural ambivalence towards differing conditions and how they might have arisen suggests that insecurity and uncertainty need now to be factored in. It is not only conditions where weight might be a factor but also those where exercise, alcohol intake and sexual practices might have a bearing.

Illness therefore joins health and fitness as reconstituted elements in Bauman's examination of the emergence of liquid modernity. Such a realisation accords with the constantly moving nature of a consumer society and gives substance to the argument that we are now living in a 'liquid modernity'. This connection is best summarised by Bauman in his earlier work, where the pursuit of fitness is identified as exemplifying the 'inner compulsion to be on the move ... the neurotic "rhyzomic", random chaotic, confused compulsive restlessness of postmodern culture with its breathtaking succession of fads and foibles. Ephemeric desires, short-lived hopes and horrid fears devoured by fears even more horrid. Postmodern cultural inventiveness may be compared to a pencil with an eraser attached; it wipes out what it writes and thus cannot stop moving over the dazzling blankness of paper' (Bauman, 1995: 119).

Fitness as a new dimension of health?

Whether valid or not, Bauman's schema for understanding the interplay between health and fitness depends to a certain degree on whether or not the concept of 'liquid modernity' has traction. Fitness may have been constructed in the period when Dennis Smith (1999) described him as the 'prophet of postmodernity' but the fact that it provides a cornerstone of Bauman's more recent collection of work on liquidity confirms that it is still an important component of his current thinking and therefore needs to be evaluated accordingly. Consequently, while, as Atkinson (2008) has pointed out, Bauman's formulation has been lumped together with the work of both Giddens and Beck in terms of their common focus on the processes of individualisation, more explicit criticism of his overall project has been limited; possibly because he still points to the inequalities and negative consequences that continue to persist in the contemporary world. In addition, the change in emphasis of his work from an espousal of the cultural effects of postmodernism to the more nuanced conditions of uncertainty promoted by liquid modernity has given him a sage-like quality not shared by the other two. Furthermore, Atkinson notes, his affinity with other radical commentators on the state of the modern world, such as Pierre Bourdieu and Richard Sennett, has also given him a degree of protection from criticism. Atkinson is not so easily satisfied that his ideas deserve exemption from criticism. In a sustained critique of Bauman's work on liquid modernity he argues that many of the flaws identified in the work of both Giddens and Beck: namely that they over emphasise the impact to which individualisation has unsettled the stability of modernity, as well as the degree to which we all live in more contingent circumstances, as is also true of Bauman's approach.

The imputed disappearance of class in modern times is the prism through which Atkinson assesses what he sees as the unfounded claims of Giddens and Beck, and now crucially Bauman. In specifically examining Bauman's views Atkinson takes issue with a crucial aspect of liquid modernity: namely the too-high emphasis on the contingency created by the effects of continual social and cultural dis-embedding, which because there is little possibility for any sustainable capacity for re-embedding creates the anxiety and insecurity central to Bauman's thinking. Bauman's vagueness about the nature of class in conditions of liquid modernity, Atkinson argues, is a case in point. When discussing the unequal effects of liquid modern processes he is inclined to utilise a binary opposition approach more familiar with Marxist categories of class conflict rather than investigate the more pluralistic viewpoint adopted by most contemporary sociologists of class including Goldthorpe and indeed Wright. This makes it easy to claim a lack of solidity in social relations and correspondingly emphasise contingency. By continually favouring dichotomous social categories in a whole number of different spheres (for example his notion of 'tourists' and 'vagabonds' in Bauman, 1998b) over more grounded descriptions he not only glosses over complex situations but is guilty of a 'spurious fluidity' (Atkinson, 2008: 13), which overemphasises 'intensified insecurity and flexibilisation of employment' (Atkinson, 2008: 14). This, argues Atkinson, leads the concept of liquid modernity to be 'an intellectual edifice constructed out of acutely unsound materials' (Atkinson, 2008: 15).

These criticisms are severe, and where Atkinson points out that internal inconsistencies regarding the potential for successful negotiation by all of the liquid modern game are compelling, however when assessed against the ideas of health and illness that are the subject of this chapter they have less purchase. Part of the reason for this may lie in the fact that notions of illness, health and fitness operate at a more cultural level, where changes in the context of health are influenced by different social pressures. The shift from a classical modernity, with its emphasis on capitalist production and its intermeshing with nation-states, created definite social forms and institutions. That these have long-term durability cannot be denied and indeed may reflect Tilly's notion of 'durable inequality' (Tilly, 1998), where exploitation and opportunity hoarding play a role in sustaining inequalities over time. However, even the processes by which this has occurred have changed over the past half century and have made problematical some of the assumptions of institutionalised inequality. The processes are much more given to flux than they have been in the past, and it is indeed the task of sociology to see the balance between what is relatively consistent and what is changing. The improved circumstances of the retired in North America and Europe is just one powerful example of how a previously marginalised and generally poor group have seen their circumstances improve for a variety of reasons;

some health related, some cultural and some quite unexpectedly economic (Gilleard and Higgs, 2000; 2005).

The fact that as Bauman points out 'quality of life' has come to replace 'a pre-occupation with self-preservation and survival' (Bauman, 1995: 78) is an important transformation of not only individual lives but also institutional structures. The welfare state is not primarily about the task of ensuring survival, instead it is now more focused on enabling a good quality of life for citizens. This end is as elusive and underdetermined as the desires engendered by consumption and consumerism. It is therefore not surprising that many of the components of the welfare state find themselves competing to provide those aspects of 'fitness' with more commercially orientated providers, and sometimes are unsure where the boundaries lie. The indeterminacy of fitness acts as a driver in a world where separate notions of illness and health are also being overwritten by medicalisation and 'healthicisation'. The capacity to successfully negotiate these discourses may be structurally overdetermined (a point acknowledged by Bauman in his *Collateral Damage*, see Bauman, 2011), but they do represent a change in the way that individuals negotiate some of the indeterminacy of what used to constitute the relatively more straightforward world of health and illness as constituted by professional and lay accounts.

To conclude, in outlining the nature of how insecurity is bound up with consumer society, Bauman, through his notion of fitness and its separation from the idea of health, offers a new template through which to view the role of health in the somatic society.

References

Atkinson, W. (2008) Not all that was solid has melted into air (or liquid): a critique of Bauman on individualization and class in liquid modernity, *Sociological Review* 56: 1–17.
Armstrong, D. (1995) The rise of surveillance medicine, *Sociology of Health and Illness* 17: 393–404.
Bauman, Z. (1988) *Freedom*, Milton Keynes, Open University Press.
——(1989) *Modernity and the Holocaust*, Cambridge, Polity.
——(1995) *Life in fragments*, London, Basil Blackwell.
——(1998a) *Work, consumerism and the new poor*, Milton Keynes, Open University Press.
——(1998b) *Globalization*, Cambridge, Polity.
——(2000) *Liquid modernity*, Cambridge, Polity.
——(2005) *Liquid life*, Cambridge, Polity.
——(2011) *Collateral Damage*, Cambridge, Polity.
Blackshaw, T. (2005) *Zygmunt Bauman*, London, Routledge.
Conrad, P. and Potter, D. (2000) From hyperactive children to ADHD adults: Observations on the expansion of medical categories, *Social Problems* 47: 559–82.
Foucault, M. (1977) *Discipline and Punish: the Birth of the Prison*. Harmondsworth: Pevegrine.
Gilleard, C. and Higgs, P. (2000) *Cultures of Ageing: Self, Citizen and the Body*, Harlow, Prentice Hall.
——(2005) *Contexts of Ageing: Class, Cohort and Community*, Cambridge, Polity Press.

Jones, I. R. and Higgs, P. (2010) The natural, the normal and the normative: Contested terrains in ageing and old age, *Social Science and Medicine* 71(8): 1513–19.

Lupton, D. (1995) *The Imperative of Health: Public Health and the Regulated Body*. London: Sage.

Marshall, B. and Katz, S. (2002) Forever Functional: Sexual Fitness and the Ageing Male Body, *Body and Society* 8: 43–70.

Outhwaite, W. (2009) Canon formation in late 20th century British sociology, *Sociology* 43: 1029–45.

Smith, D. (1999) *Zygmunt Bauman: Prophet of postmodernity*, Cambridge, Polity.

Tilly, C. (1998) *Durable Inequality*, Berkeley, CA, University of California Press.

3 Jürgen Habermas

Politics and morality in health and medicine

Gemma Edwards

German critical theorist, Jürgen Habermas, is generally known for offering a rather dense and abstract theory of modern capitalist society. There continue to be moves however to apply his concepts in ways that relate to concrete issues in empirical research. A promising branch of this 'applied turn' has put Habermas's ideas to use in research on health and medicine. Here, his concepts have led to critical engagement with issues of medicalization and medical expertise, doctor–patient interactions and clinical practice, and collective action around health in the public sphere (see Scambler, 2001).

This work has shown that Habermasian theory can be a valuable asset in research on health and medicine. This is because his concepts of 'system', 'lifeworld' and 'colonization' focus attention on issues of a political and moral nature and raise questions of real concern, like: 'does the doctor know best?'; 'how far should patients be involved in their treatment?'; and 'how should knowledge about the causes, treatment and prevention of illness be constructed?' The political issues raised relate to power and democratic practices, whilst moral debates centre on how to ensure recognition and human dignity in medical settings.

In fact, raising these kinds of issues confirms the relevance of Habermas's theory of modern society for health today. In many ways he is able to prefigure current conflicts between expert and lay approaches to health, and the moral controversies that arise therein. The evidence for this comes largely from looking at the collective struggles of health movements in the public sphere. It is social movements, after all, that politicize and remoralize health issues. The struggles of health-related 'new social movements' in particular suggest that the concerns raised by Habermas continue to be a source of both moral debate and political mobilization.

I suggest here, therefore, that Habermas has been used to good effect to understand conflicts surrounding the growing power of medical expertise in everyday life, and the collective struggles of social movements to 'reclaim' health. A key part of Habermas's argument, however, is the (related) growth of the state and the market into areas of everyday life, but there have been relatively few attempts to look at this process in relation to health (with some rejecting its relevance, Fredriksen, 2003). I argue here that this is a symptom of the conceptual problems that belie Habermas's distinction between 'system' and 'lifeworld' more generally. I suggest that there is a need to rethink 'system' and 'lifeworld' in order to apply Habermas's theory to conflicts surrounding the state, market and health. It is in the context of public health services, I contend, that the battle lines between everyday communicative practices on the one hand, and money and power on the other, are drawn and fought over today.

The chapter proceeds as follows: first I outline Habermas's concepts of 'lifeworld' and 'system' and the conflict between them, pointing to the way in which he prefigures a set of moral and political concerns relevant to health and medicine. Second, I look at how these conflicts play out in the collective struggles of health social movements. In the latter part of the chapter, I present a conceptual critique of 'system/lifeworld' in order to consider colonization and resistance in public health services today.

The lifeworld: health in everyday life and the patient perspective

Health is a central aspect of everyday life. The importance of health is often brought to our awareness in circumstances where it is taken away. Ill-health has a basic influence not only on the body, but on how a person lives, how they think of themselves, and how they relate to others. Personal identity, lifestyle and social relationships are therefore shaped by the experience of being healthy, or not. When a person becomes ill, for example, they have to renegotiate their sense of self (as an 'ill' person), their way of life (within the constraints of illness), and their relationships to others (such as family and friends who are very much implicated in the experience of illness) (Kelleher, 2001). The personal experience of illness (as the sufferer or their loved one) therefore leads to a great deal of subjective knowledge referred to as 'lay knowledge' (Williams and Popay, 2001). Lay knowledge surrounds the impact of illness on the whole person (mental as well as physical), what makes the person feel better or worse, and how medical treatments work in the context of people's daily lives.

Health is therefore a key element in what Habermas (1987) called the 'lifeworld'. At a basic level, the 'lifeworld' refers to everyday life and the perspective that people have of the world that arises out of it. Everyday life takes place in particular socio-cultural contexts. It consists of relationships and interactions with others that operate on the basis of shared cultural meanings, understandings and assumptions. In the course of everyday interactions with others – which happen primarily through a shared language – people invoke and thus (much of the time anyway) reproduce these cultural meanings, understandings and assumptions. Personal identities are also formed and reproduced through interactions with others (Mead, 1934). We gain a sense of who we are as an individual, for example, by having our 'self' reflected back to us through the 'looking glass' (Cooley, 1902) provided by others.

The lifeworld, then, consists of three key elements: culture (shared knowledge, meanings, assumptions), society (social relationships) and personality (personal identities) (Habermas, 1987: 135). In the medical literature, Habermas's concept of the lifeworld has been taken to refer to the patient's perspective on illness that arises from these three elements: from their particular cultural context (knowledge and way of life); from their social relationships (within families and communities); and from their individual viewpoint (including the effect that being ill has upon their sense of self). Mishler, for example, defines the 'voice of the lifeworld' as 'the patient's contextually-grounded experiences of events and problems in her life' (Mishler, 1984: 104).

The lifeworld, and its three key elements, are created and reproduced through the medium of linguistic communication – or what Habermas (1987) called 'communicative interaction'. Communicative interaction is a key concept in Habermas's theoretical framework. When people interact communicatively they engage in speech aimed at understanding one another. The process of communicative interaction involves jointly constructing the definition of the situation, negotiating and renegotiating the meaning of the situation, and the process of argumentation (putting forward reasons, listening to those of others and proceeding on the basis of the 'better argument') (Habermas, 1987: 145). Cooperation in everyday life depends therefore upon communicative interaction. Habermas states:

> In communicative action participants pursue their plans cooperatively on the basis of a shared definition of the situation. If a shared definition of the situation has first to be negotiated ... the attainment of consensus can itself become an end ... Participants cannot attain their goals if they cannot meet the need for mutual understanding.
>
> (Habermas, 1987: 126–27)

It is also important to note that through argumentation, communicative interaction enables people to make aspects of their lifeworld – which are normally assumed (Schutz, 1974) – the subject of debate. Through communicative interaction, 'taken for granted' aspects of life can be placed under the moral spotlight. In the 'public sphere', for example, Habermas (1989) argues that citizens remoralize issues of concern through their discussion and debate and put them on the political agenda. People have not always been able to reflect upon the background assumptions of their lives in this way, however. In this respect, communicative interaction is a trait of the 'modern' lifeworld, produced by a process of 'rationalization' in social life more generally.

The rationalization of society had been interpreted rather negatively by Habermas's predecessors, like Max Weber (1978), who saw it as the spread of 'instrumental rationality' (i.e. more and more areas of life becoming subject to calculation, control and the drive for profit, like for example the spread of bureaucracy and its associated 'iron-cage'). However, for Habermas, rationalization also involved a process similar to what Weber called 'disenchantment'. As traditional societies gave way to modern ones, myth and religion lost their power to structure reality for people in ways that could not be open to challenge. This is a positive form of rationalization, according to Habermas, because it opens up to question aspects of a lifeworld 'taken for granted'. Furthermore, the only way to answer the questions raised is through communication aimed at understanding.

In the modern lifeworld, for example, people have to 'achieve' a consensus on moral issues through discussion and debate because other grounds (like tradition) have been lost. In an open process of dialogue, the people affected explain how they feel, give reasons for their position, listen to the reasons of others and come to mutual decisions about what they ought to do. Decisions made under such conditions, Habermas (1996) argues, can be said to be moral and justifiable. Moreover, in communicative interaction people must reach decisions on the basis of 'the better argument' alone, and (in ideal situations at least) must not be influenced by other agendas, like those relating to money and power (Habermas, 1987: 145).

In the medical literature, it has been suggested that the interaction that takes place between the doctor and patient in a consultation should at least strive to be 'communicative' in this manner. The definition of illness and a course of treatment should, for example, be negotiated through an open dialogue that is not influenced by the power of medical expertise. Doctor and patient should construct a mutually acceptable definition of 'the problem', and come to a consensus about how it should be treated. Often this 'ideal' is not lived up to, however. Research has shown that by enforcing their 'expert' opinion, doctors subordinate the patient's lay knowledge, and details about their wider life context (Mishler, 1984; Scambler, 1987; Barry et al., 2001; Greenhalgh et al., 2006). Subsequently, 'the lifeworld is rarely heard or acknowledged by the physician' (Leanza et al., 2010: 1888). When the doctor dominates interaction in this way, the communication becomes (in Habermas's language) 'distorted'. In real terms, distorted communication between the doctor and patient means that the patient may leave the consultation feeling like the doctor was not listening to them, or did not really understand the nature of their illness. Consequently, the patient perspective – rooted in everyday life and experience – can be discounted or underplayed.

In this respect, the 'voice of the lifeworld', Mishler (1984) argues, is dominated by the 'voice of medicine'. Mishler (1984) bases this observation on his research into consultations in hospitals and private practices in the US. The dominance of the voice of medicine has been connected with important moral concerns in medicine. These include patient liberty, particularly when it means that treatment options are limited or imposed (Scambler, 1987). It has also been linked with accusations of 'inhumane' medical care, which fails to recognise the patient as a unique individual (Mishler, 1984). Whilst the word 'inhumane' is perhaps too strong to describe clinical practices that are dominated by medical experts (Barry et al., 2001: 491), communicative interactions are nevertheless positively associated with more 'patient-centred' and democratic healthcare. We will return to these conflicts later, but first it is necessary to consider Habermas's concept of 'system' in order to understand where this 'voice of medicine' comes from.

The system: modern medicine and the expert perspective

Habermas argues that there are some areas in society that do not operate on the basis of communicative interaction and are therefore outside of the 'lifeworld'. Specifically, interactions involved in economic activities and the activities of nation-states have evolved on quite different principles. The key difference is that they are rooted in 'instrumental' rather than 'communicative' action. We can revisit Weber's theory on rationalization to illustrate this point. Weber (1978) argued that as capitalist societies develop, life becomes increasingly rationalized in the sense that more areas are opened up to principles of calculation, control and the drive for profit ('instrumental rationalization'). Furthermore, to achieve success, these areas are orientated to an interest in scientific knowledge and expertise that can address their technical concerns, like how best to master and control processes (Habermas, 1971). Two areas have evolved according to these principles: the capitalist market, and the modern nation-state. These areas – coordinated through instrumental/technical action and scientific expertise – are what Habermas (1987) refers to as 'the system'.

Habermas (1987) argues that as the economy and state develop into a complex instrumental/technical system, they become increasingly divorced from communicative practices and thus 'uncoupled' from the lifeworld. The system, for example, is more interested in the most efficient means to an end, rather than ends in themselves, and in success and control, rather than understanding and consensus. This is reflected in the value placed upon expert scientific knowledge, technology and (often statistical) evidence in shaping dominant assumptions and action in the system. The lifeworld is also viewed through this expert lens as a subsystem in itself, which provides important resources for the overall system, like motivation and commitment (which have to be rooted in everyday life). From a system point of view, the lifeworld is another object to be mastered and controlled by system experts.

This image of the 'system' can be a useful way to think about the nature of modern medicine (Scambler, 2001; Barry *et al.*, 2001; Fredriksen, 2003). Modern medicine, in contrast to health, is part of the 'system' rather than the 'lifeworld'. It consists of a body of expert medical knowledge shaped by science and technology. It has an instrumental orientation towards the successful treatment of ill bodies, and a technical orientation towards the mastery and control of biological processes (Barry *et al.*, 2001: 489). It approaches bodies primarily as objects for medical intervention, and in doing so abstracts individuals from their wider lifeworld context. For example, patients are talked about as numerical codes that specify their conditions (H1N1 patient, for example), are charted, administered and reduced to health statistics. Lifeworld problems are also turned into 'technical' ones. Fredriksen draws upon the example of psychiatry's approach to grief counselling, where he argues that 'what was, and in effect still is, a personal and relational crisis shaking the foundations of our existence is transformed into an objective situation in need of manipulation' (Fredriksen, 2003: 292).

Modern medicine is also delivered to the public primarily through state-bureaucratic institutions, like GP surgeries, hospitals, mental institutions, care homes and the like. Market principles, too, have been introduced into aspects of healthcare, for example by the privatization of public health services, and the commercialization of health problems and treatments (leading to big profits in pharmaceuticals). Equally, modern medicine is fond of scientific expertise and not particularly open to lay knowledge. Instead it sticks to its dominant ways of defining, treating and preventing disease drawn from expert knowledge. This 'biomedical model' of illness (Kelleher, 2001) is generally not up for debate by the patient. Modern medicine is therefore an institution steered by bureaucracy, the market and the power of medical expertise, but not, primarily, by communicative interaction.

Whilst the 'voice of the lifeworld' denotes the patient's experiences, knowledge and perspectives drawn from everyday life, the 'voice of medicine' therefore denotes the dominant biomedical model of illness and the perspective of medical experts (Mishler, 1984). The 'voice of medicine' seeks to control the body-as-object, whereas the voice of the lifeworld seeks an approach to illness that shows an understanding and recognition of the context of everyday life. Conflict, then, seems inevitable.

The conflict between system and lifeworld: colonization and medicalization

The kind of conflict that Habermas is interested in does not simply arise from the existence of two different perspectives and ways of doing things. There is nothing inherently problematic, for example, about the instrumental/technical action of the system. In fact, Habermas (1987) acknowledges that the development of complex instrumental/technical systems guided by expert knowledge has brought about many improvements and advantages for modern society. Unlike his critical theory predecessors, he does not lay the blame at the door of instrumental rationalization itself (see Adorno and Horkheimer, 1944). Indeed, modern medicine is a prime example of the progress that can be achieved by the drive to control nature through scientific expertise. So where does the problem lie?

Habermas suggests that modern capitalist societies are characterized by social conflicts that 'arise along the seams between system and lifeworld' (Habermas, 1987: 395). More specifically, these conflicts surround where the 'boundaries' are to be drawn between the instrumental/technical system on the one hand, and the communicative practices of everyday life on the other (Habermas, 1996a: 363). It is Habermas's contention that in modern societies the system has a tendency to grow, and keep on growing, until it extends its reach back into the lifeworld. This means that the economy (the capitalist market and its drive for profit) and the nation-state (with its legal and bureaucratic forms of power) start to 'take over' increasing areas of life that were previously thought to be beyond their reach, like for example the private life of the family, and activities relating to education and health. Current concerns around the commercialization of culture and identity, the marketization of education, and the privatization of the national health services, are good examples of this.

These processes are problematic because the instrumental/technical way of doing things (that is characteristic of the system) replaces everyday communicative practices. As discussed earlier, communicative practices are essential for reproducing everyday life, including cultural knowledge, social relationships and personal identity. When communicative interaction is replaced by instrumental/technical action (and, furthermore, when expert knowledge erodes lay knowledge), there are 'pathological' side effects for culture, society and personality – in short, for the lifeworld itself. As a result, people experience a 'loss of meaning' in their daily lives and what Habermas (1987) calls 'cultural impoverishment'. It is this kind of conflict between 'system' and 'lifeworld' that Habermas sees as characteristic of modern society, and he terms it the 'colonization of the lifeworld by the system':

> The thesis of internal colonization states that the subsystems of the economy and state become more complex as a consequence of capitalist growth, and penetrate ever deeper into the symbolic reproduction of the lifeworld.
> (Habermas, 1987: 367)

It is important to note that Habermas (1987) believes that the conflicts surrounding colonization have replaced those surrounding class and labour as the key conflicts in modern capitalist society. He explains this shift with reference to the growth of the welfare state. He argues that the welfare state represented a victory for the working class and labour movements, who fought the government for a range of assurances and benefits that would protect workers from the worst effects of capitalism (like unemployment and poverty). What they did not foresee, however, was that, once established, the welfare state would keep on growing and would introduce a new set of conflicts around communication and culture. For example, the welfare state extended state bureaucracy and law into more and more areas of the lifeworld, a process that Habermas (1987) refers to as 'juridification'. Through social policy it sought to govern and reshape ways of life, social relationships and personal identities. In particular, through policies relating to health and social care, the welfare state increasingly turned people into 'clients' of state bureaucracies.

In fact, the specific example that Habermas gives of colonization is social and health policy (1987: 395). Through state intervention in the lifeworld, care for groups like the elderly and the mentally ill, for example, have been removed from families and communities and provided instead by state institutions and medical experts. People are encouraged through this new set up to view health and social care as an 'individual right' that has to be claimed by the individual, and results in them being 'administered' by the state. In the process of removing health and social care from everyday contexts, people's identities and relationships become redefined by the system and potentially problematic. The change in roles and expectations initiated by the intervention of the state can also break down existing family and community support for those in need of care. Habermas argues that:

> ... the individualising definition of, say, geriatric care has burdensome consequences for the self-image of the person concerned, and for his relations

with spouse, friends, neighbours, and others; it also has consequences for the readiness of solidaristic communities to provide subsidiary assistance.

(Habermas, 1987: 362)

Colonization, then, points to the way in which health is increasingly removed from everyday life and administered through state bureaucratic institutions ('juridification'). This is the image of colonization that Habermas (1987) most definitely had in mind. Colonization can also point, however, to the way in which health is increasingly commercialized and privatized by the introduction of the market. Habermas (1987) calls this process 'commodification', although he has much less to say about it in the way of examples. It could refer, however, to the way in which health provision is increasingly shaped by neo-liberal health policies in the present context, a process that includes the growth of both money (the market) and (political) power (Scambler and Kelleher, 2006). By and large, however, colonization has not been talked about in these terms in the medical literature. Indeed, some have rejected the relevance of state/market growth for health (Fredriksen, 2003). Instead, emphasis has been placed upon colonization in terms of the (related) growth of medical expertise in everyday life.

In this respect, it has been suggested that the 'medicalization' of society is a prime example of the 'colonization' of health by the system (Scambler, 2001; Barry et al., 2001; Fredriksen, 2003). 'Medicalization' refers to the increasing dominance of medical experts over the way in which health and illness are defined, approached and treated in society. It also refers to the way in which people become increasingly reliant upon professional healthcare services and technological/drug interventions, to the extent that they are transformed into the 'worried well' (Fredriksen, 2003: 288). Expert medical advice even pertains to issues as basic as how much you should weigh (Crossley, 2004).

It has been suggested, therefore, that cases where 'the voice of medicine' dominates over 'the voice of the lifeworld' are prime examples of 'colonization' (Mishler, 1984; Scambler, 1987). The distorted communication between doctors and patients in medical consultations, discussed earlier, is not just a conflict over two differing perspectives, but a case of 'the colonization of the lifeworld' by expert scientific knowledge (Barry et al., 2001; Greenhalgh et al., 2006).

The colonization of health by the expert 'voice of medicine' points, then, to a range of political and moral issues. These include questions like: 'how far should the power of medical experts dominate knowledge and understanding of health?'; 'What role should science and technology play in defining illness and shaping treatment?'; 'How far should the "biomedical model" be open to debate by patients?'; 'Can the social interactions that take place within medical settings ensure the recognition of patients as individuals?'; 'And to what extent is the "whole person" considered in medical treatment?' Colonization does not only raise these questions, however. According to Habermas (1981), it also initiates collective struggles on the part of social movements to address them in the public sphere. How far, then, do the concerns of health movements reflect the kind of moral and political issues prefigured by 'the colonization of the lifeworld by the system'? And to what extent can their activism be understood in Habermasian terms?

Collective action around health and medicine: 'new social movements' against colonization?

Habermas (1987) argues that the political and moral concerns created by 'the colonization of the lifeworld' directly lead to the mobilization of social movements. Social movements (as collective actions around issues of public contention) instigate critical public debate about the 'growth of the system' (Habermas, 1981), and become the vehicles through which technical questions are repoliticized and remoralized in the public sphere. Habermas (1981) calls contemporary social movements that respond to colonization 'new social movements'. This is to distinguish them from the 'old' social movements which were class based and mobilized around issues of labour and political rights. The 'old' social movements engaged far more overtly in political confrontations with the state over material resources and their distribution. New social movements, on the other hand, respond to 'the colonization of the lifeworld' by operating on more cultural and personal terrain. In the loose-knit, informal networks of everyday life (like friendship groups), they challenge the dominant definitions, knowledge and assumptions of the system and emphasize the value of personal experience (Melucci, 1989). They seek to defend and reclaim personal and collective identities, and base collective action in these identities (Melucci, 1989). In this sense, 'new social movements' are a different kettle of fish compared to labour and political rights movements.

Habermas's examples of 'new social movements' include those that challenge the way in which social and health policy turn people into 'clients' of state bureaucracy. Here he talks about anti-psychiatry and self-help groups (Habermas, 1981). The first wave anti-psychiatry movement of the 1960s, for example, challenged the way in which psychiatry defined certain problems as 'mental illness' and treated them through incarceration in state-bureaucratic institutions, like mental hospitals (Crossley, 1999). Anti-psychiatry activists established self-help groups in which personal experience was privileged as a form of understanding problems, and where people could construct more positive images of themselves. Personal and collective identities were 'reclaimed', for example, through participants defining themselves as 'survivors' rather than 'patients' of psychiatric institutions (Crossley, 2006). Arguments were also made against the use of certain medical treatments for mental illness – like electric shock therapy – claiming not only that it did not work, but that it was morally wrong and undermined human rights.

Analysis of health movements today has moved away from viewing resistance as a simple response to the ever-growing net of state bureaucracy. Nevertheless, concerns about the way in which people are turned into 'clients' of health services, run by medical experts, persist. It has been suggested, for example, that a range of health movements today are concerned with challenging the dominance of expert medical science.

Mental health groups (Rogers and Pilgrim, 1991), disability movements (Oliver, 1990), movements around HIV/AIDS (Epstein, 1996), and self-help groups for diabetes sufferers (Kelleher, 1994) have been analysed in these terms as 'new social movements' that resist the way in which expert knowledge 'takes over' personal experience and understandings of health. Political activism arises, for example, from the desire to challenge dominant medical discourse about illness, or question the science behind it. Personal identities can become politicized when:

> ... institutions of science and medicine fail to offer disease accounts that are consistent with individuals' experiences of illness, or when science and medicine offer accounts of disease that individuals are unwilling to accept, people may adopt an identity as an aggrieved illness sufferer and even progress to collective action.
> (Brown et al., 2004: 55)

Brown et al. (2004) refer to the movements that contest medical science as 'embodied health movements' and draw upon Habermas's concept of 'new social movements' (in part) to understand them. These 'embodied health movements' draw upon people's personal experience of health problems to challenge medical assumptions about cause, treatment and prevention. The US environmental breast cancer movement is one of their examples. It sought to bring to the attention of scientists the environmental hazards that activists believe are linked with breast cancer. It also argued that treatment for breast cancer should take account of the 'whole woman' and her social existence, warning of the dangers of approaching the breast purely as an object for medical intervention and control. They associate the latter approach with morally contestable treatment options, like the (now outlawed) practice of performing mastectomies without consent (Brown et al., 2004).

Allsop et al. (2004) similarly suggest that 'health consumer groups' are 'new social movements' rooted in personal experience of illness, which try to 'change perceptions of professionals and public' (Allsop et al., 2004: 741). These groups perhaps more explicitly mobilize around the 'client' role, although in the current neo-liberal climate, patients are moreover 'consumers' of health services. Health consumer groups are formed by the users of health services in order to gain recognition of their needs (for example, relating to childbirth), or to construct positive personal identities out of their experiences of living with conditions (ranging from cancer and arthritis to mental health). Interestingly, Allsop et al. argue that health consumer groups develop an idea of the 'expert patient' (2004: 745) in order to challenge expert medicine.

Habermas's concept of 'colonization' does seem useful therefore for understanding the moral and political concerns of contemporary health movements about the growing power of medical expertise in everyday life. His concept of 'new social movements' fits particularly well in this respect with the concerns of 'embodied health movements'. The medical literature (for a second time), however, tends to concentrate first and foremost upon struggles surrounding the growth of medical expertise, and less explicitly so upon struggles initiated by the growth of the state and the market in health. Although the two are related, money and political power nevertheless raise other types of concerns as well.

Scambler and Kelleher (2006) for example look at how the campaigns of health movements seek to reveal the connections between ill-health and the context of people's everyday lives, including the hazards that exist in the local environment (like pollution from cars, toxic waste, water pollution, pylons, etc.). These hazards are not only poorly recognized by expert science, but they also relate to the 'colonization' of the physical environment of the lifeworld by state and global capitalist agendas (Scambler and Kelleher, 2006). Indeed, the close connection between the state, economy and health is made clear in the alternative globalization movement, which associates health risks with the global drive for profit, state-sponsored environmental destruction and economic deprivation (Crossley, 2012). Environmental social movements, like Greenpeace and Friends of the Earth, also make these connections and see health as a central issue in their campaigns (Scambler and Kelleher, 2006: 228).

It would also be wrong to uncritically suggest that 'embodied health movements' fit seamlessly within Habermas's account. In fact, they complicate matters somewhat because they do not straightforwardly campaign to 'keep the system out' of the lifeworld. The environmental breast cancer movement, for example, aimed to get medical experts to intervene in the issue and wanted to produce alternative expert knowledge by gaining a seat at the scientific table (Brown *et al.*, 2004). The desire for a dialogue between lay and expert knowledge is particularly likely in cases where health issues are experienced as problematic by people in their everyday lives, but are not well recognized by science (like chronic fatigue syndrome and gulf war syndrome, for example) (Crossley, 2012). Health movements are, then, involved in 'blurring boundaries' (Brown *et al.*, 2004: 63–64) and not just 'policing boundaries' – to use Habermas's phrase – between modern medicine and everyday life. Scientific evidence and knowledge are very important to health activists, and not simply a target of attack. The current public debate in the UK about whether to vaccinate all children under five from swine flu, for example, has not only involved parents contesting expert medical opinion with personal experience, but attempts on the part of the public to collate scientific and statistical evidence to support the alternative case.

Health social movements suggest, therefore, that whilst Habermas's ideas of 'system', 'lifeworld' and 'colonization' may help in understanding the nature of contemporary concerns around health, there are also problems with his account. Health movements do not simply fight 'to keep the system out', but seek in some cases to cross the boundaries between system and lifeworld. This, in itself, is suggestive of the fact that 'system' and 'lifeworld' are intermeshed in ways more complex than Habermas suggests. There is a need to look again at what 'system' and 'lifeworld' really mean. Indeed, I suggest that if Habermas's ideas are to be useful for looking at the relationship between the state, the market and health (as well as the power of medical expertise), then we need to rethink 'system' and 'lifeworld' in more subtle terms.

Rethinking 'system' and 'lifeworld': colonization and resistance in public health services

In what way, then, is the distinction that Habermas draws between 'system' and 'lifeworld' problematic? As we have seen, Habermas bases this distinction on a division between instrumental/technical action and communicative action. He then categorizes areas of life as 'system' or 'lifeworld' on this basis. For example, he sees health and education as dependent on understanding and consensus and therefore part of the 'lifeworld'. Work, on the other hand, is his prime example of instrumental and technical action, and is part of the system (Habermas, 1974). This distinction has been hotly contested in social theory (Giddens, 1982; Honneth, 1982; Edwards, 2007). Work, for example, is a key site for the reproduction of personal identities, especially gendered ones (Fraser, 1989).

In fact, the division between 'work' and the 'lifeworld' (or 'work' and 'interaction', as Habermas, 1974, draws it) leads to a particularly tricky issue when applying Habermas's ideas in contemporary welfare state societies, where health and medicine are primarily organized as 'services' (like, for example, the NHS in the UK). Even though the existence of health as a service could be deemed an example of a first wave of 'juridification' in Habermas's terms (where state bureaucracies 'take over' areas of everyday life), it does also mean that much of the debate surrounding health and medicine takes place today in relation to health services. The concern here is not just about the way in which health services are run by medical experts, but the way in which they are shaped by money (the market) and (political) power.

Public health services create a tricky issue for Habermas because they evade simple categorization as either 'system' or 'lifeworld', and are instead situated between the two. Offe (1985), for example, talks of the contradictory nature of service work, which requires 'normatively based substantive rationality' rather than 'technical rationality', because what it produces are concrete 'uses' rather than 'monetary profit' (Offe, 1985: 138–39). Habermas appears to accept Offe's point when he states that 'labour seems to be shifting into domains which are unfamiliar which activities modelled on industrial labour, which rather demand communicative interaction with persons' (Habermas, 1986: 142–43). Employees of the health service, for example, are clearly asked to work within the dominant 'biomedical model' and according to the instrumental practices laid down by their employers and the state (i.e. caring for people efficiently and cost effectively). Nevertheless, the nature of their work (the 'caring for people' bit) means that they cannot simply adopt an instrumental/technical approach, but need to interact in ways aimed at understanding and consensus, too.

As a consequence of these competing demands, employees become caught up in tensions created when the communicative practices involved in doing their job clash with the dominant medical model and expectations (e.g. pressure to use established approaches to treatment over alternative therapies, pressure to cut costs, to cut waiting lists, to succeed in league tables and so forth). These kinds of tensions are characteristic of the public sector more generally (Edwards, 2009). In fact, the position of the health service as caught *between* 'system' and 'lifeworld' helps to understand the kind of conflicts that arise there. This point has been made clear in studies of maternity care. Maternity care has been seen as a good example of where mutual understanding, consensus and cooperation are, what Habermas would call, a 'functional necessity' (Habermas, 1987: 369). Drawing upon interviews with midwives in Ireland, Hyde and Roche-Reid (2004) look at the way in which they are torn between the competing demands of providing care communicatively (catered to the individual woman's experiences, needs and choices), and working in accordance with the practices imposed by the 'technocratic system of obstetrics'. Midwives inevitably find it difficult to juggle both 'system' and 'lifeworld' agendas. This is because, as Offe states:

> the criteria of rationality of the organisation (effectiveness, efficiency, control, standardization ... etc) clash with the autonomy and flexibility requirements *(of service activities)*.
>
> (Offe, 1985: 107)

The idea of health as a service therefore means that it is necessary to rethink what 'system' and 'lifeworld' really mean. It does not make much sense to talk of areas of society – whether the health service, schools or work organizations more generally – as either 'system' *or* 'lifeworld'. 'System' and 'lifeworld' are instead better thought of as a battle between two different ways of doing things – two distinct 'logics of action' – that exist everywhere in society (Edwards, 2009). Indeed, this makes sense, argues Fraser (1989), 'if the real point' is that communicative practices are 'morally superior'. If this is the case, then it should be desirable for workplaces and political institutions to operate on communicative principles as well (Fraser, 1989: 135). This is arguably the case in the health service, where communicative interaction is necessary to ensure that questions of a moral nature, which (necessarily) arise at work, are not simply transformed into 'technical' issues for management control.

This conceptual critique of 'system/lifeworld' repositions Habermas's ideas in a way that makes them useful for understanding the nature of conflict in public health services. It is here, for example, that tensions between everyday health practices on the one hand, and the state and market on the other, are primarily played out today. The health service can, for instance, be subject to an *intensification* of bureaucracy and market relations, which signify *further* attempts to 'colonize' health by money and power.

Whilst concerns over bureaucracy in the health service continue to persist, it is the growth of the market that is producing most conflict and debate at the present time. For example, recent government proposals in England and Wales (in January 2011) argue that the NHS needs to 'modernize', largely by introducing more of a market. This will be done by increasing the number of private sector providers, who will compete over price with the NHS. These proposals are coupled with moves away from centralized, state-run services and towards putting power and control more firmly in the hands of GPs and 'patient-consumers'. 'Commodification', then, is to be the present-day remedy for 'juridification'.

Doctors and nurses have expressed 'extreme concern' over these changes. Six health unions, the British Medical Association and the Royal College of Nursing, for example, articulated these in a letter to *The Times* newspaper (17 January 2011), arguing that market competition in the health service would put concerns of cost (the 'system') over those of patient care and quality (the 'lifeworld'). The colonization of the health service leads to concerns, therefore, not only for 'clients', 'consumers' and 'citizens' of the state, but for 'employees' of the state as well. It also has the potential to reignite the kind of labour and union struggles that Habermas had left behind.

Conclusion

Embodied health movements – and collective struggles around public health services – share in common a desire to resist the 'colonization of the lifeworld by the system'. To this extent, Habermas's theory of modern society is highly relevant and decidedly useful for thinking about the nature of moral and political conflict in health and medicine today. In particular, his concepts of 'system', 'lifeworld' and 'colonization' seem to capture something of the contemporary concern around the growing power of medical expertise in everyday life. This does not mean, however, that his concepts can be used without qualification. The 'lifeworld' – that is subject to colonization – is not an area of life that lies outside of the system, and must defend itself from its ever-growing reach. It is more complicated than that. The 'lifeworld' does not exist apart from the 'system', and never has. Rather, the state and the economy constitute the lifeworld in the first place (Honneth, 1981), and always have.

Our everyday lives – culture, social relationships and personal identities – are, for example, fundamentally shaped by the state and the economy, and, furthermore, by science, technology and expert knowledge. The contour of the battle between these elements is anything but predictable. Social movements in the past have fought, for example, to get the state to intervene *even more* in everyday life (as struggles *for* a national health service attest). And embodied health movements today fight to get the attention of medical experts so that what they feel from their personal experience can become scientifically known and validated. Health movements do not, therefore – straightforwardly at least – strive to 'get the system out' of the lifeworld ('decolonization'), or to completely replace expert scientific knowledge with lay knowledge ('reclaim').

What they do involve, however, are challenges to the instances where system 'ways of doing things' (instrumental/technical) come into conflict with communicative 'ways of doing things' and create problems for people in their everyday lives (as clients, consumers and citizens of the state, but as employees of the state too). The problem is not primarily with using scientific knowledge and expertise as a means to an end, but with failing to debate what those ends should be. Equally, the problem is not with science and technology controlling and manipulating biological processes, but with forgetting to ask when it is, and *is not*, appropriate for them to do so. By the same token, the problem is not with the state and the market in health, but with money and power displacing communicative practices by putting concerns of administration and cost before those of human life. In this situation, health-related new social movements, and collective struggles around public health services, are important because they bring back communicative interaction through the very way in which they challenge and debate (Scambler and Kelleher, 2006). They make it clear to government, public and academics alike, that questions about what happens in areas of life, like health, are first and foremost questions about politics and morality.

References

Adorno, T. and Horkheimer, M. (1944) *Dialectic of Enlightenment*. London: Verso.
Allsop, J., Jones, K. and Baggott, R. (2004) 'Health consumer groups in the UK: a new social movement?' *Sociology of Health and Illness*, 26(6): 737–56.
Barry, C., Stevenson, F., Britten, N., Barber, N. and Bradley, C. (2001) 'Giving voice to the lifeworld. More humane, more effective medical care? A qualitative study of doctor–patient communication in general practice', *Social Science and Medicine*, 53: 487–505.
Brown, P., Zavestoski, S., McCormick, S., Mayer, B., Morello-Frosch, R. and Gasior Altman, R. (2004) 'Embodied health movements: new approaches to social movements in health', *Sociology of Health and Illness*, 26(1): 50–80.
Cooley, C. (1902) *Human Nature and the Social Order*. New York: Charles Scribner's Sons.
Crossley, N. (1999) 'Fish, field, habitus and madness: the first wave mental health users movement in Great Britain', *British Journal of Sociology*, 50(4): 647–70.
——(2004) 'Fat is a sociological issue: Obesity rates in late modern, "body-conscious" society', *Social Theory and Health*, 2: 222–53.
——(2006) *Contesting Psychiatry*. London: Routledge.
——(2012) 'Social Movements and Health' in Monaghan, L. & Gabe, J. (eds.) *Key Concepts in Medical Sociology*. London: Sage.
Edwards, G. (2007) 'Habermas, Activism and Acquiescence: Reactions to Colonization in UK Trade Unions'. *Social Movement Studies*, 6(2): 111–30.
——(2009) 'Public Sector Trade Unionism in the UK: Strategic Challenges in the face of Colonization', *Work, Employment and Society*, 23(3): 442–59.
Epstein, S. (1996) *Impure Science: AIDS, Activism and the Politics of Knowledge*. Berkeley: University of California Press.
Fraser, N. (1989) *Unruly Practices: Power, Discourse and Gender in Contemporary Social Theory*. Cambridge: Polity Press.
Fredriksen, S. (2003) 'Instrumental colonisation in modern medicine', *Medicine, Healthcare and Philosophy*, 6: 287–96.
Giddens, A. (1982) 'Work and Interaction', in J. Thompson and D. Held (eds.) *Habermas: Critical Debates*. Cambridge, MA: MIT Press.
Greenhalgh, T., Robb, N. and Scambler, G. (2006) 'Communicative and strategic action in interpersonal consultations in primary healthcare: A Habermasian perspective', *Social Science and Medicine*, 63: 1170–87.
Habermas, J. (1971) *Toward a Rational Society*. Boston, MA: Beacon Press.
——(1974) 'Labour and Interaction', in J. Habermas, *Theory and Practice*. London: Heinemann.
——(1981) 'New Social Movements', *Telos*, 49: 33–37.
——(1986) in P. Dews (ed.) *Autonomy and Solidarity: Interviews with Jürgen Habermas*. London: Verso.

——(1987) *The Theory of Communicative Action volume II*. Cambridge: Polity.
——(1989) *The Structural Transformation of the Public Sphere*. Cambridge: Polity.
——(1996) *Between Facts and Norms: Contributions to a Discourse Theory of Law and Democracy*. Cambridge: Polity.
——(1996a) 'The Normative Content of Modernity', in extracts from *The Philosophical Discourse of Modernity*, XII, pp. 336–67, in W. Outhwaite (ed) *The Habermas Reader*. Cambridge: Polity.
Honneth, A. (1981) 'The Dialectics of Rationalization: An Interview with Jürgen Habermas, by A. Honneth, E. Knodler-Bunte and A. Widmann', *Telos*, 49: 5–31.
——(1982) 'Work and Instrumental Action', *New German Critique*, 26: 31–54.
Hyde, A. and Roche-Reid, B. (2004) 'Midwifery practice and the crisis of modernity: implications for the role of the midwife', *Social Science and Medicine*, 58: 2613–23.
Kelleher, D. (1994) 'Self-help groups and their relationship to medicine', in J. Gabe, D. Kelleher and G. Williams (eds.) *Challenging Medicine*. London: Routledge.
——(2001) 'New social movements in the health domain', in G. Scambler (ed.) *Habermas, Critical Theory and Health*. London: Routledge.
Leanza, Y., Boivin, I. and Rosenberg, E. (2010) 'Interruptions and Resistance: A comparison of medical consultations with family and trained interpreters', *Social Science and Medicine*, 70: 1888–95.
Mead, G. H. (1934) *Mind, Self and Society*. Chicago: University of Chicago Press.
Melucci, A. (1989) *Nomads of the Presents: Social movements and individual needs in contemporary society*. London: Hutchinson.
Mishler, E. (1984) *The Discourse of Medicine: Dialectics of Medical Interviews*. Norwood, NJ: Ablex.
Offe, C. 1985 *Disorganized Capitalism: Contemporary Transformations of Work and Politics*. Cambridge: Polity.
Oliver, M. (1990) *The Politics of Disablement*. Basingstoke: Macmillan.
Rogers, A. and Pilgrim, D. (1991) 'Pulling down churches: accounting for the British Mental Health User's Movement', *Sociology of Health and Illness*, 13(2): 129–48.
Scambler, G. (1987) 'Habermas and the power of medical expertise', in G. Scambler (ed.) *Sociological Theory and Medical Sociology*.
——(2001) (ed.) *Habermas, Critical Theory and Health*. London: Routledge.
Scambler, G. and Kelleher, D. (2006) 'New social and health movements: Issues of representation and change', *Critical Public Health*, 16(3): 219–31.
Schutz, A. (1974) *The Structures of the Life-World*. London: Heinemann Educational Publishers.
Weber, M. (1978) *Economy and Society*, Los Angeles: University of California Press.
Williams, G. and Popay, J. (2001) 'Lay knowledge and the concept of the lifeworld', in G. Scambler (ed.) *Habermas, Critical Theory and Health*. London: Routledge.

4 Luhmann's social systems theory, health and illness

Barry Gibson and Olga Boiko

When Niklas Luhmann set out to construct a systems theory of society he produced what is arguably one of the most extensive and comprehensive projects to date in sociology. His theory has been described as a series of 'theory pieces' (Hornung, 2006). The theory is at one and the same time a theory of societal differentiation, social systems, observation, distinction and societal semantics. Providing an adequate summary in such a small space is therefore a difficult task.[1] This chapter begins with a brief introduction to Luhmann's social systems theory. The idea is to provide an account of the main elements of his approach, after which we hope to provide a brief outline of the main approaches adopted by Luhmann for the analysis of social systems. Luhmann's work on health has yet to be translated and so we are faced with the perennial problem of reading Luhmann, and this is related to the accessibility of his principal ideas. The chapter then goes on to provide a critical evaluation of the ways in which Luhmann has been applied to the field of health and illness before demonstrating how his ideas can be used to explore a common problem: that of the emergence of communication about dentine sensitivity and quality of life.

Luhmann's social systems theory: a brief introduction

Luhmann's social systems theory is known for his attempt at a complete revision of sociology. Luhmann borrowed many concepts from cybernetic theory, systems theory, Spencer-Brown's laws of form, theoretical biology and from differentiation theory (Hornung, 2006). Luhmann was also resolutely anti-humanist. Indeed, as Hornung (2006) has stated, there is no one theory at the heart of Luhmann but many 'theory pieces'. This is because his work was always a science in process. It is the combination of influences, the borrowed language and the developmental nature of his project that frequently makes reading Luhmann a difficult task. When reading Luhmann one has to be aware that he was often addressing conceptual problems in sociology, problems that social systems theory had to solve and problems that are particular to the ongoing empirical analysis he was undertaking. An additional complication was that much of the work that he references, and he enjoyed referencing extensively, is printed in German. A consequence of this is that it is difficult to trace the sources of his ideas, to check his interpretation of those sources and to clarify meaning. Reading Luhmann is therefore not easy and this task is not made easier by the fact that much of his work remains inaccessible to those without a good command of German. This is why the introductory texts outlined in the notes to this chapter are so useful and important.

Society for Luhmann is composed of communications and nothing but communications. Luhmann frequently joked that society was actually 'less than the sum of its parts'; in other words it is something that does not include people but is rather something that happens *between* them. Society, in his perspective, occurs in the spaces between people rather than encompassing and including them. It derives its principal dynamics, not from human beings, but from patterns of communication and how these are organised. Such patterns of communication historically have coalesced around recurrent problems. The central claim of Luhmann is that the communications themselves eventually organised into specific kinds of systems that subsequently separated themselves into specialist spheres of communication. One of the central problems that Luhmann studies is how such separation happened and what were its many consequences.

As stated above some writers have described Luhmann's work as containing several 'theory pieces' (Hornung, 2006, King and Thornhill, 2003). One of these theory pieces involves Luhmann's reinterpretation of Parsons's view of society as being composed of a series of functionally differentiated systems. In contrast to Parsons, Luhmann's theory has been described as a functional structural theory instead of a structural functional theory (King & Thornhill, 2006). By reversing the order of function and structure Luhmann's innovation was to see structures and functions as essentially contingent. The fact that structures emerge is almost a mystery. There are problems that require solutions and are continually the subject of communication. Eventually these communications develop a condensed structure; an organised complexity; a system. Such systematic communications eventually specialise to the point where systems separate or differentiate themselves. The history of modernity is, in part, a history of how such differentiation has occurred. It is this self-determining aspect of Luhmann's social systems that gives his theory one of its many peculiar characteristics. Specifically this involves the concept of 'autopoiesis'.

Luhmann's use of autopoiesis was adopted from the work of two Chilean biologists Humberta Maturana and Francisco Varela, and it refers to the process whereby living organisms reproduce themselves by producing the parts that produce themselves (Maturana and Varela, 1980). In other words living systems are characterised by their self-referentiality. The theoretical innovation of autopoiesis is not a novel innovation in the sense that other philosophies and cosmologies have used similar concepts (Moeller, 2006). Such systems produce themselves through the reproduction of their elements and are therefore self-constituting. An autopoietic system is organisationally separated from its environment by a barrier. This barrier is permeable in the sense that matter and energy can pass through it from the environment. Such exchanges are essential for the system to survive. Upon passing through the barrier, however, the matter or energy is changed to become part of the system (King, 2009). Such systems continually reproduce their parts;

indeed they do so by constantly changing those parts so that the system remains even though it is constantly changing. In applying these ideas to society, Luhmann was in some way able to overcome the kind of criticisms levelled at Parsons's structural functionalism (for being too static); it enabled him to produce a much more 'organic' account of social structure.

The copying of autopoiesis into social systems theory had a number of consequences. As has already been indicated, autopoietic systems are organisationally closed but energetically open. Such social systems are circular in their organisation and are therefore insensitive, i.e. they cannot be changed very easily. A key consequence of this conception of society and social systems is that it becomes extremely important to focus on the relationship between each system and its environment. Each system must distinguish itself from its environment. The environment is both undifferentiated and system specific. What this means is that there will be things the system cannot observe but nonetheless remain in the environment of the system, and there will be an environment that the system constructs almost exclusively for itself. In other words the system sees an indeterminate environment and it also sees itself in a 'relevant environment' (Pelikan, 2007).

Controversially, autopoietic social systems have their own dynamics; they cannot get their principal dynamics from people. They are of course dependent on people for their existence; in this respect they are energetically open. Luhmann used the term 'structurally coupled' to describe the relationship between people and social systems. The idea was best described in the following quotation taken from *Political Theory in the Welfare State*:

> Human beings, concrete individual persons, take part in all social systems. But they do not enter into any of these as determinate parts themselves nor into society itself. Society is not composed of human beings, it is composed of communications among human beings.
>
> (Luhmann, 1991: 30)

Society therefore at some point in history developed specific spheres of communication established around specialist functions. At this point society became primarily characterised as being functionally differentiated. No longer were people classified according to their position in a social hierarchy as they had been in the previous stratificatory society, although that form of social organisation did not go away either (Luhmann, 1990b). Indeed whilst relations of inequality are an important feature of society they are not its determining relation. The argument goes in Luhmann that the newly emerging communication systems eventually achieved a degree of freedom from each other and indeed from the individuals whom they were dependent on for their existence. Moeller (2006) and King (2009) both describe this very neatly when they state that society is in fact composed of multiple communicative realities. There is no privileged position from which to view society, no unifying worldview behind society, despite what Habermas and others might think. But what are the systems that we are speaking of?

The functional systems that Luhmann was most concerned with were the economy, the legal system, politics, the mass media and art. He wrote about education and health but these short books have yet to be published in English. In addition to these specific systems there were other forms of communication that were quite general but which have not become systems; such forms include ecological communication, risk communication and morality, amongst other things (Luhmann, 1989, 1993). It is important to understand that systems and indeed all forms of communication operate on the basis of 'distinctions'. The inspiration for this was derived from Luhmann's adaptation of Spencer-Brown's *Laws of Form* (Spencer-Brown, 1969).

Distinctions operate on a number of levels. When communication occurs the observation 'draws a mark', that is it marks out what is to be included in communication and what is to be left out. Whilst this might seem to represent the return of binary oppositions this is simply not true. In fact there is an in-built bias contained within all distinctions. What is inside the boundary of the distinction is the 'valued' side. What this means is that the chain of communication will 'connect' on the basis of this value. This requires some illustration. A simple object is indicated when it is called and everything else that is outside of the basic distinction is left unobserved (see Figure 4.1). In the example in Figure 4.1 we have a chair indicated and what is outside of this is an indeterminate other, the world. The world is composed of a virtually infinite number of objects that can be made the subject of communication. There are however more complex distinctions such as concepts.

Concepts occur when the other side of the distinction is restricted or called. In Figure 4.1 the concept of gender is composed of female and male. These two indications subsequently restrict communication to the theme of gender, and simultaneously gender communication becomes thematised around the competition between male and female. In this instance female is valued over male, as it might have been in the past in early forms of feminism. The analysis does not stop there however. There are more complex 'second-order' distinctions. The classic case is given of the difference between government and opposition (Figure 4.1).

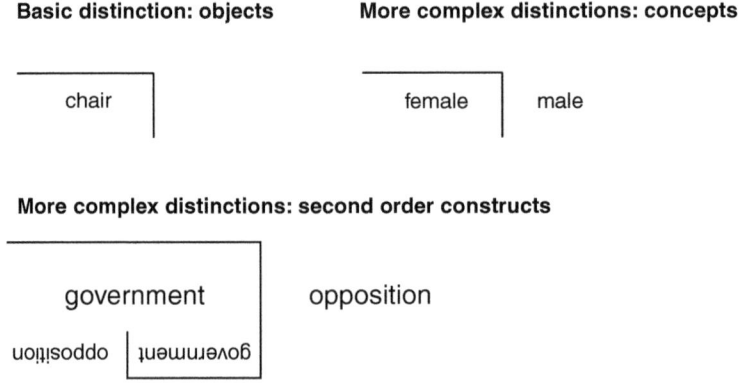

Figure 4.1 The use of distinctions in Luhmann's social systems theory

Second-order distinctions fold back on themselves and produce a re-entry of the distinction into itself. So whilst the government has an opposition that is outside of itself the government will also have an opposition within itself. The ruling elite within government are opposed by others who are nevertheless in the same government. The evolution of such complex forms of communication gives modern society its particular character. Before continuing the introduction of Luhmann's theory, a short pause to explore how some of these ideas have been applied to health is in order.

The application of Luhmann to the study of health and illness

When we talk about health systems in this approach we are talking about how communications about health and illness are organised and actualised. Specifically, we should focus on how chains of communication can happen and ask why this is the case. Studies that draw on Luhmann will therefore be studies about how health communication is organised. Luhmann never wrote a specific monograph on health systems although he clearly assumed they existed (Pelikan, 2007). He did write several short papers on the topic all of which remain in German (Luhmann, 1983a, 1983b, 1990a). There are several places where the work of Luhmann has been applied to the study of health systems (Michailakis and Schirmer, 2010, Pelikan, 2007, Gregory et al., 2005, Boiko et al. 2011, Gilson, 2003, Meyer et al., 2008). Others have related their work to Luhmann in the study of health and illness, but Luhmann has not been central to their analyses (Murphy and Pilotta, 1987, Gibson et al., 2005, Osborne, 1993, Reznik et al., 2007, Birenbaum-Carmeli, 2004, Lonardi, 2007).

The most detailed application of Luhmann to health systems in general we could find has been outlined by Pelikan (2007). Pelikan (2007) begins by exploring the application of Luhmann's social systems theory to an alternative perspective on health status measurement. The first section of his chapter therefore explains how the system environment distinction can be applied to understanding health as a polycentric phenomenon, centred on the interactions between three separate systems and their respective environments. He then goes on to explain the specific mechanism of autopoiesis and how it can be used to understand health as a basic property of systems (Pelikan, 2007). For our purposes however the most interesting aspect of his analysis is reserved for his application of Luhmann's approach to the analysis of health in modernity. Specifically Pelikan (2007) states that this approach results in two questions: are there specific systems specialised in processing problems of human health in society, and secondly have specific sciences related to health developed?

Luhmann clearly assumed there was a health system and that its code was sick/healthy or health and illness, with illness being the valued side of the distinction (Luhmann, 1983a, 1983b, 1990a). Luhmann's use of health versus illness seems to have come under some criticism in the German literature, and this has led to others going on to propose a broader code, that of hindering and promoting health (Glotzer et al., 1995, Bauch, 1996, 2000). In this work we discover more and more of the details of how Luhmann's theory is to be applied. We find out for example that the definition of the binary code is crucial because it sets the boundaries of the system. In the case of the health system, by opting for illness vs. health or ill vs. healthy, Luhmann was clearly arguing for a specific limitation to the health system. By criticising this code Pelikan (2007) and others (Glotzer et al., 1995, Bauch, 1996, 2000) argue that the domain of the health system is much broader than Luhmann envisaged. So for example Pelikan (2007) argues that the code could in fact be the presence vs. absence of physical illness or suboptimal vs. optimal physical positive health. These codes become important when we start to consider that considerable efforts are made in society to promote and manage the health of populations.

Pelikan (2007) went on to ask if a specific function system for public health had evolved or, alternatively, if public health communications had emerged as a set of several separate but nonetheless interrelated communications within different function systems such as science education and politics. It was argued that there was considerable evidence that society had engaged with public health; for example, we have had the emergence of a new expert called the 'public health' expert. This development on its own is not, however, enough to constitute a system in its own right. Nonetheless for Pelikan (2007) even if there wasn't a specific social structure for public health but rather sub-structures and function systems dedicated to public health, what seems to have emerged is a specific semantic for public health. This semantic, it is argued, has allowed the generation of public health to be considered within the sub-divisions of other function systems.

Pelikan (2007) continues his analysis by arguing that the binary code for public health could be formulated as the presence or absence of pathogenic risk factors in the environment. Therefore, in order to change the unhealthy behaviours of individuals and populations, the programme of public health had moved towards health education and media campaigns. There is also under development a specific area for public health knowledge, so for example we have journals and conferences dedicated to public health. This begs the question: what keeps public health together as a social unity? Looking at this problem, Pelikan (2007) argued that semantically there was a shared code, a variety of shared programmes and these had facilitated the accumulation of shared knowledge. Indeed perhaps it would be more appropriate to call public health a new, albeit state-sponsored, social movement; a movement that seeks to ensure and improve the health of populations. Indeed this movement has had some success in initiating and using research, law, education and the mass media systems to plan, implement and legitimise its policies and programmes (Pelikan, 2007).

Pelikan (2007) goes on to demonstrate how public health experts in fact operate in the spaces between organisations dedicated to health; in so doing they enable the coupling of decisions between organisations at the same time. They often frequently work with many groups at once to enable multiple effects across function systems over time. This has led to a form of intensive referencing of the involved systems to each other. So, for example, public health education, public health mass media communication, public health politics and public health research all reference each other (Pelikan, 2007). For Pelikan (2007) this begged the question: why has public health not been as successful as clinical medicine or the other social movements for health in modernity? Pelikan (2007) goes on to compare and contrast clinical medicine to public health. For him the principle difference between the two was that clinical medicine was orientated to treating the actual ill-health of single individuals whereas public health on the other hand was orientated to avoiding the future 'possible ill-health' of 'abstract populations'. Public health had to intervene into social living conditions, lifestyles and the environment of populations. It had to intervene into the functioning of society itself and therefore depended heavily on social interventions, social conditions, processes and behaviours. Luhmann's approach is especially useful because it helps us focus on society as a series of functionally differentiated communication systems (Luhmann, 1995). Seeing these systems as separate and organised according to their own codes with their own boundaries enables us to begin to unpick the complexity of activity at the heart of health movements such as that associated with public health. This view of public health contrasts to the view that it is a purely state-sponsored activity, rather it involves a whole series of communications, not necessarily coordinated across different poly-contextual 'realities'.

Luhmann's systems theory clearly argues that it is an error to see the health of the public as simply a matter for state control. Indeed in his perspective the relationship between state and society is reformulated. The state should not be seen as a technology for central planning and control; indeed Luhmann was very critical of this technocratic perspective. Rather than mistaking the relationship between state and society as the model for the whole society, it was important to realise that functional differentiation had occurred, that there were processes ongoing to solve problems within each of the function systems and that, thankfully, these were not under the control of the state (Arato, 1994). Indeed the problem with political power was its ability to be purely arbitrary, causing disturbances throughout society almost at whim; we only need to look at the sheer volume of changes that occur when governments change to realise that we should be grateful that the arbitrary power of the state is limited in some way (indeed as Luhmann stated, the state often had to set limits on itself otherwise it would destroy the process of differentiation).

For Luhmann the idea of a civil society, largely in opposition to government, is in fact decomposed by his model of differentiation. In other words there was no core to society. Rather society was split into separate functional social systems and this had obvious consequences for the activity and nature of public health. The rest of this chapter seeks to illustrate how society has in fact found solutions to problems that remain almost completely outside of state control. Luhmann's sociology has a whole series of analytics that can be applied. It has been argued, in fact, that his approach would be best described as being divided into a series of 'analytics' (Andersen, 2003).

Luhmann's 'analytics'

Luhmann's social systems theory is an explicit focus on communications and as a consequence there are a number of analytical strategies that can be used. These have been summarised by Andersen (2003) (see Table 4.1). The analysis provided by Pelikan (2007) is very much an analysis of the health system and the possibility of a public health system. In many ways the analysis provides us with a complex exploration of the health system set alongside an analysis of the semantics of public health. There are other analytics that can and indeed have been deployed

Table 4.1 Luhmann's analytical strategies*

Analytical strategy	General question	Examples
Form analysis	What is the unity of the distinction? And which paradox does it establish?	In what way are organisations systems that communicate through the form 'decision'? And which paradoxes does this form establish?
Systems analysis	How does a system come into being in a distinction between system and environment? How is the systems boundary of meaning and autopoiesis defined?	In what way does the politicisation of the organisation become apparent in the internal construction by the organisations of their environment so that they not only construct the environment as market but also as political public?
Differentiation analysis	How are systems differentiated? What is the similarity in the dissimilarities of the systems? What are the conditions, therefore, of the formation of new systems of communication?	In what way does the politicisation of the organisation challenge their internal form of differentiation and force them to institutionalise internal reflections of themselves as closed communication (for example through so-called 'ethics officers')?
Semantic analysis	How is meaning condensed and how does it produce a pool of forms, that is, stable and partially general distinctions available to the systems of communication?	How is what health 'means' condensed with respect to environment, human rights, ethics, animal welfare, health and prevention, into the concept of the 'socially responsible corporation', and bring about new conditions for corporate communication?
Media analysis	How are media shaped? How do they suggest a specific potential for formation?	In what way does the politicisation of the organisation mean that the organisation is no longer only supposed to form the medium of money, but is also expected to form a number of other communicative media such as power, information and morals? In what way does this change the conditions of the organisation from homophony to polyphony?

*Reproduced with kind permission from Andersen (2003: 93).

to study the phenomenon of health in society. The most directly popular of these has been form and semantic analysis.

Form and semantic analysis was deployed in the work of Boiko et al. (2011) who explored forms of communication in dental encounters. Boiko et al. (2011) challenged approaches that sought to divide communication in medical systems into 'system and lifeworld'. 'Pure binary oppositions', appeared to be less central to the dynamics of communication. Indeed, it seemed that both dentists and patients could circulate in their observation of the problem by drawing on a series of well-established distinctions, for example, in the case of a look–feel semantics exploring the difference between sensations and clinical signs (Boiko et al., 2011). Both patients and dentists could be seen to observe the mouth in terms of feelings and knowledge of clinical signs. There was no simple dichotomy between the system and the lifeworld, or at least it did not seem to be that central to the communications as they unfolded in their work.

As we have said earlier, the perspective of Luhmann's social systems theory tells us to pay close attention to how systems relate to their environments. In particular we should observe closely which system is communicating. So, for example, if we are reading a scientific paper we would expect its primary purpose to be scientific communication, its primary distinction, the distinction that will predominate, will be on the relative truth or falsity of something. Likewise when a patient refers to something about their health or their illness we are primarily observing communications in a social interaction, either a research interview or if we are watching medical consultations as an interaction between doctor and patient. Not all communication is a social systemic communication however. Sure, at times when patients do communicate, they are participating in medical systemic communications, at other times they will not be. In short not every communication participates in a social system, yet nonetheless all communication is part of society (King, 2009). Communication enters into consciousness in the form of thoughts and both social and psychic systems share the same medium. That of meaning:

> Communications cannot penetrate consciousness except as thoughts. In the social sphere thoughts are able to enter only as communications which convey meaning, which can be understood or misunderstood ... we could say that using the medium of meaning, people as conscious systems, and society as a communication system form a necessary environment for one another.
> (King, 2009: 60)

In other words meaning ties psychic and social systems together. Luhmann developed these ideas further by, for example, drawing on Parsons's notion of symbolically generalised media of communication. According to Luhmann (1995) symbolically generalised media 'use generalisations to symbolise the link between selection and motivation, that is, represent it as a unity' (Luhmann, 1995: 161). Pelikan argues that for the medical system this is the system of differential diagnosis (2007: 89). In order for it to work as part of a system, symbolically generalised media must have 'symbiotic mechanisms', that is it must have practices that link the medium to the human body. In the case of the medical system there are at least three and possibly more such mechanisms: surgery, pharmacy and radiology (Pelikan, 2007). We would like to explore this further by taking the example of how everyday communications about a common health problem, i.e. dentine sensitivity, might be understood from the perspective of systems theory.

Form analysis and the paradoxes of dentine sensitivity

This section aims to continue our introduction of the methodology of form analysis and to show its application to the analysis of healthcare communication. Our goal is to further demonstrate its use in discussing narratives on dentine hypersensitivity.

As we have seen form has been described as a basic distinction between two sides divided by cloven or a 'slash' (day/night) (see Figure 4.1). Andersen (2003) outlines after Luhmann (1993) three different kinds of form: objects, first-order concepts and second-order concepts. The original sources that informed Luhmann's perspective on different types of distinction or form ranged from formal logic to meaning constructions[1].

The evolution of forms from object (i.e. table/not table) to first-order forms (i.e. married/single) and then second-order forms (i.e. risk/danger) was particularly important for this empirical analysis. Indeed the methodological discovery of systems theory has been that a simple binary logic of first-order forms is not developed enough for dealing with the complex phenomena of modern societies. It was for this reason that Luhmann argued for the functional necessity of second-order forms, which were more sensitive to the polyphony of meanings. For example, the distinction medical professional/patient surpassed the level of first-order observation in contemporary healthcare. In effect it lost the simple dichotomy as patients have been enabled to access professional knowledge and expertise of their conditions. The distinction medical professional/patient nowadays could easily be observed as a more intricate second-order form. Likewise, the second-order form – health/illness – has become exposed to greater complexity and reflexivity. Such distinctions have resulted in paradoxes associated with health – people's experiences of health could not be subject to logical divisions; two sides of health and illness stopped being mutually exclusive and the experience of health and illness frequently co-exist (Pelikan, 2007). To Luhmann, observations in complex social systems have emerged so reflexively that communications can use and re-use previous distinctions. This process of 'folding back in' was called the operation of re-entry and is described in Figure 4.1 in relation to the second-order distinction of government and opposition. Here, the paradox of form became apparent: one had to start by dividing and making distinctions to discover the opposite: the similarities and interdependence. In other words, an attempt to eliminate or distil one side of the form only reinforced a 'self-referential' back loop.

Forms, and especially, second-order forms, therefore, have the strategic goal of making sense and communicating about the world. Consequently, form analysis, designed in the recent study of dental encounters (Boiko *et al.*, 2011) sought to deploy this logic in dealing with real time communications. It was found that participants could not only think by differentiating between things, they also communicated their distinctions, and by doing so created meanings of the events, symptoms and health conditions. Having this proposition in mind enabled the application of form analysis to be applied to 'real-time' communications around oral health. The methodology of form analysis was developed to distinguish first- and second-order forms from verbal exchanges. It was found that there were a great number of distinctions, indeed every utterance has the potential to give rise to a basic form – in this respect the method allowed creating procedures for an inductive analytical process. In line with other qualitative methods of data analysis (grounded theory, thematic and framework analysis, etc.), the rule of thumb has been to abstract from utterances into generalisable categories (forms). The point of difference, however, resided in the fact that the forms, in contrast to categories or themes, were based on distinctions and also based on the authentic utterances of the participants in communication. For instance, always/might be was one of the examples of a (probabilistic) first-order form extracted from dentist–patient communications, which enabled dentists and patients to explore what will and what may happen concerning the behaviour of the patient's denture (Boiko et al., 2011).

As far as the analytical procedures were concerned two basic rules of connectivity and repetition were applied to the analysis of data. This involved reading the data line by line and marking out sequences of words that were connected over time and in a logical manner achieving the sense of distinction. Often words appeared in an adjacent position in communications. Repetition implied that, even when two words did not follow one another, they recursively appeared in different places and related to similar issues. Forms were then tested on their complexity, reflexivity and possible paradox of re-entry to establish first- or second-order level of observation. Taking another example from the previous study, the dentist's communication: 'It might look a little bit sore and you'll feel sorry for yourself', gave rise to the complex form look/feel (Boiko et al., 2011). Additionally, our study aimed at abstracting even higher order forms called semantics, which reflected the clinical system functionality. Look/feel eventually was observed and analysed as one of the semantic forms functionally significant to the dentistry.

Dentine hypersensitivity: a case study

The current study of the experiences of dentine hypersensitivity used the same methodological insights and procedures of form analysis. This study was a follow-up of a larger project supported by GlaxoSmithKline and aimed at exploring the everyday impacts of dentine sensitivity on everyday life (Gibson et al., 2010, Boiko et al., 2010). The findings of this previous work suggested that dentine sensitivity (i.e. sensitive teeth) presented differently among the study participants. While some people disclosed the chronic character of the condition with significant impact on their daily functioning and activities, others reported less impact and were not prepared to treat it as a disease. In these latter interviews participants shared different strategies of self-management, most commonly avoidance (of food) and adaptation (changing eating patterns) strategies. Importantly, the use of sensitive toothpastes varied between and within the group of chronic sufferers and occasional 'victims' of sensitivity. Some of these variations in narratives prompted the need for follow up interviews. Our presumption was that Luhmann's approach may encourage a further insight into the experiences of dentine sensitivity, related health identities and also allow us to explore the dilemmas of self-management and toothpaste consumption. We felt that form analysis might be useful in understanding the paradoxes of the condition, in particular, in exploring how participants were able to draw the distinction between sensitivity as both a health and an illness condition.

The qualitative study discussed in this chapter received the ethical approval from the ethics committee of the University of Sheffield. Interviews were conducted with 16 participants (seven males and nine females), recruited from the general population by snowballing (dentine sensitivity is a widespread condition, one in four or one in three members of the adult population will admit to or are diagnosed with sensitivity). All participants were interviewed twice with a two-week time period. The first interviews aimed at expanding on people's experiences of the condition, their health beliefs and health identity. The second round of interviews concerned the use of toothpaste, self-care and consumer strategies of participants. The interviews were further studied using the method of form analysis. Distinctions were identified on the basis of the connectivity and repetition of utterances within and between interviews. These distinctions composed the basis of first- and second-order forms of communication about dentine sensitivity. We were also interested in establishing, for each form, the unity of the distinctions and the paradoxes they established (see Table 4.1). The search for second-order forms resulted in the analysis of 16 forms, six of which are discussed here in some depth.

Describing the sensitivity pain: sharp/short

Clinical studies conventionally classified dentine hypersensitivity among undifferentiated pain-evoking oral conditions, and for a few decades dentists treated it as an enigma (Harris and Curtin, 1976). Our earlier qualitative study identified no less than 22 nominations of the sensations attributed to the pain of dentine sensitivity. It also uncovered the very complex character of sensitivity associated with differences in intensity, duration, tolerability and unpredictability (Gibson *et al.*, 2010). Yet, most people articulated the episodes of short and sharp pain in teeth as the key qualities of the condition. This result was confirmed by form analysis in the current study. A number of homogeneous first-order distinctions such as shooting/stops, quick/uncomfortable, intense/instantaneous, intense/not constant were extracted from the interview data. However, the search was for an overarching second-order form that could encompass these experiences. The following quote demonstrates such a form extracted from the data:

> Usually, it's relatively instantaneous and I sort of have a little aftershock for a little while, it's quite sharp and short pain, it's just they are sensitive, as soon as I take away whatever is causing it.
>
> (S1.4)

The form sharp/short encompassed a range of basic descriptions of pain and was studied as the generic form in relation to other distinctions. It was for this reason (and for fulfilling repetition and connectivity criteria) that the form received the status of a second-order form. The form also corresponded with clinical definitions of the condition as associated with sharp, short pain (Dababneh et al., 1999). The individuals' narratives corresponded well with a clinically approved definition of the condition as a sharp, short pain in teeth. In other words, form analysis lent support to our understanding of dentine sensitivity as reflecting intermittent pain episodes. The prominent paradox of sensitivity pain, therefore, could be explained by the short horizon of physiological response, which made it possible to tolerate and cope with the pain of high intensity. However disturbing and uncomfortable the nature of the pain was – 'brain freeze', 'nails on the blackboard', 'needles', 'burst inside' – the sensation had often lasted seconds, usually conditioned by the exposure to a stimulus: cold drinks and food, hot drinks and food, toothbrushing and cold air. In Luhmann's terms, even though the sharp pain was selected as the first side of the form, it was short so that the other side (short) penetrated the first side (sharp), opening up a paradox of re-entry. Following from Luhmann's analytics as outlined by Andersen (2003) in Table 4.1, there are two questions we need to address. What is the unity of the distinction and which paradox does it establish?

The unity of this distinction at the heart of dentine sensitivity is that of transient pain (Melzack, 1973). The paradox is that although the pain is 'sharp' it is 'short', delimited temporally but painful nonetheless. It is a limited experience that has a limited impact but it hurts. The nature of the pain, as we found out in the interviews, was communicated as an infrequent and unpredictable event. This analysis lends support to the idea that there is a paradox of sensitivity. This paradox, we would argue, explained why many interviewees did not seek any cure for their condition. What makes this a paradox however?

The clash of shortness and sharpness as communicated in dentine sensitivity make it what it is. Now this is not a 'logical paradox' but is what Luhmann refers to as an 'entangled hierarchy' (Luhmann and Behnke, 1994). This hierarchy is the entangled nature of the relationship between the temporality of pain and its sharpness. This form, the difference between the shortness and sharpness of sensitivity, has consequences that bind the condition to a particular description. It is short and sharp, and not a major life problem.

In our interviews this description was provided both by those who had not yet spoken with their dentist about their sensitivity and those who had consulted a dentist. Therefore, the form of these sensations as they were expressed by our participants was not always a reflection of any particular systemic communication. This does not mean such descriptions have not become systematised in the past. To the contrary, we know for example that dentine sensitivity is defined in the scientific literature as 'a short and sharp pain' (Canadian Advisory Board on Dentin Hypersensitivity, 2003). In many respects this description has been copied into the health system and used. In this respect the form of such descriptions has in fact become a medium for the health system. It is a form that has been repeated so often to dentists and dental scientists over time that it is now accepted as a defining characteristic of dentine sensitivity.

Is this a case of the health system dominating or simply the health system observing how dentine sensitivity can be communicated? We cannot provide a detailed answer to that question here because it would involve exploring the historical semantics of dentine sensitivity. However, what we can suggest, from the perspective of Luhmann's systems theory, is that the fact that dentine sensitivity can be communicated as a 'short sharp pain' is evidence of a link between the health system and the consciousness of patients. This link is not a case of system dominance, but is in fact a link where the form of a patient's experiences described also forms part of how the health system understands sensitivity. It is also important to realise that this form restricts what dentine sensitivity is, and even though it is restricted by definition this is nonetheless still an important achievement of communication. It tells us what dentine sensitivity is and indeed helps us to see it as a restricted problem that we can manage ourselves.

Everyday impact: avoid/stop and tolerate/accept

Pain aside, dentine sensitivity caused other impacts on individuals' daily lives. These impacts were secondary to physiological reactions and related, in particular, to eating and drinking practices, and to some degree, to talking, socialising and toothbrushing. The interviewees often talked about their own strategies of adaptation, such as avoidance of food, either of changing their diet or the changing ways of food preparation and consumption. It might have been a total ice-cream abstinence; yet, at times it led to significant deprivation and withdrawal – in their words: 'I can't eat my breakfast', 'healthy things like carrots or cucumber, things that are cold and hard', 'cut it out completely'. Such 'aggressive' secondary impacts of sensitivity pain were extracted from their narratives and summed up in the first-order distinctions: don't eat/gets better, stop/helps, impacted/cut off and affect/stop. Since eating was affected the most and in a fairly common way by dentine sensitivity, we were forced to suggest that food restrictions were in fact a second-order form avoid/stop: the quote below represented its modified version (avoiding/stopped eating):

> It is about things that are very sweet that were causing intense pain on the first bite and I was avoiding those, as a result. So my wife makes fudge in the catering company and it's very sweet, 50 per cent sugar in fudge, and that I was finding on the first bite so I've stopped eating that.
>
> (S1.8)

The paradox of the form avoid/stop contained the idea that participants had to subjugate to the external force associated with pain-evoking foods, so that they were less able to cope with the impacts of dentine hypersensitivity other than through a blunt withdrawal from such foods. Avoidance became the paramount response to some products so that certain foods underwent a redefinition as taboos. The decision to stop consuming them was exacerbated by the fact that food and eating rendered a basic human necessity – some had to avoid 'pleasant' eating experiences.

Other forms of the passive, 'reflex-like' adaptation were also apparent in the narratives, leading to the second-order form tolerate/accept. In contrast to the form avoid/stop this form subsumed the experiences of endurance in continuing the normal activities despite occasional discomfort. Typical first-order forms were: put up with/used to, eat/put up with, adapt/accept. Similar logic applied to the second-order form tolerate/accept:

> I'm the kind of a person who tolerate things so when I get these sensations I'll just accept it, you know what I mean, it is one of those things.
> (S1.7)

The form tolerate/accept described the management of impacts through painstaking strategies. Like the form avoid/stop it invoked the paradoxes of unaided, adaptive management of dentine hypersensitivity. The dilemma was this: avoid or endure. It was interesting that tolerating impacts was often associated by the interviewees with ignorance ('stubbornness'), stoicism and habitual discomfort. Additional adaptation strategies such as changing eating patterns, toothbrushing practices (no rinsing, rinsing with warm water), putting a scarf over one's mouth, etc., similarly provided only a partial sense of control over the condition.

Considered in the quality of life context, these distal symptoms (Armstrong et al., 2007) fall into the category of the secondary impacts of dentine sensitivity. It goes along with a general debate on impairing or disabling conditions of the other diseases and their reconsiderations in the recent classifications of the WHO. Functional impacts on activity and participation have been legitimised within a growing awareness of quality of life issues in health and medical systems. Systems theory gives considerable currency to this too; for example Michailakis and Schirmer (2010) illustrate how the recognition of extended biopsychosocial understanding of illnesses not only changed the medical system but created disturbances for the political system.

Our analysis of second-order forms avoid/stop and tolerate/accept, and the paradoxes of adaptation associated with it, points to the importance of the unity of their distinctions. According to Luhmann, 'if one tries to observe both sides of the distinction one uses at the same time, one sees a paradox' (Luhmann, 2002: 101). This implies reflexivity in folding and unfolding both sides – so that paradoxically avoidance may actually turn into deprivation (stopping) in consuming food, and tolerance could hardly make up for acceptance of pain and discomfort. This is why we would like to call this the paradox of adaptive management, a paradox that can be partially solved by accounting for the impact of severity. Occasional deprivation corresponded with occasional pain, marrying the paradox of adaptation and the paradox of pain. Perhaps, individuals with dentine sensitivity considered themselves as maintaining health identity rather than experiencing chronic illness?

Habitualising the condition: habit/lifestyle

Central to a health identity framework, our analysis of dentine hypersensitivity highlights the dilemmas of health and self-management. Interviewees stressed the personal significance of their choices and adjustments to the condition. Most of the practices of adaptation described above – not to mention cutting fruit into bits, biting small pieces, warming up foods, cooling their tea down and other food modifications – all these became natural to their lives. In fact, most people normalised all the fuss around the condition, they justified their new habits without rethinking it in terms of drastic lifestyle changes: subconsciously/lifestyle, question it/just live, habit/living. Therefore, the generic second-order form habit/lifestyle appeared in one of the interviews:

> I think there are a lot of people who get it worse than me, it really is to the point they have to change their lifestyle, what they eat because of it, now I wouldn't say I change what I eat. I think I've got into a habit of living with it rather than trying to prevent it.
>
> (S1.15)

As the quote suggested there was a certain resistance to admit to lifestyle changes, while the notion of the habit was found comforting. 'Habit' meant the normalisation to health, health condition rather than illness condition: 'because habitually I don't eat things like that with my teeth' (S1.8). Confirming that 'humans are very adaptable' (S1.9), the interviewee accepted and adjusted to the condition, giving it a slight degree of notice. Many agreed that they 'got used to it' in their daily routines, either subconsciously or with some awareness of the changes in lifestyle (more often among chronic sufferers). Others tried to ignore the impact by integrating sensitivity into the context of their lives, a normalising response to, at times, a disabling condition. Sensitivity in teeth became integral to their lives and to their health identity. The paradox habit/lifestyle was essentially the one of health identity that underpinned minimising the impact and normalising dentine hypersensitivity as a health condition. The literature on health identity lends some support to this idea, for example, Fox and Ward (2008) argued for everyday practices of maintaining health identity ('what people do') rather than for cherishing a 'healthy' self-image. It could be positive actions for heath like walking and swimming, but it could also be adjustment practices like toothbrushing with lukewarm water and other actions discussed above.

Again we have two implications for the paradox and for systemic communication. They both suggest that the paradox of health identity is much more intricate than it seems. Because lifestyle is generally subject to moral judgements in both the public and health systems domain, the individuals in our interviews were more likely to resist selecting the side of lifestyle. Lifestyle implies a conscious health-related choice, while habits were individual preferences and ways of doing things. Habits could be ill-founded, yet, not necessarily far-reaching and deeply rooted in identity. Indeed, Michailakis and Schirmer (2010) showed how lifestyle choices turn into a burden for systems, especially where lifestyles are allegedly unhealthy, such as smoking and overeating.

As for the systemic interpretation, the medical system would not be concerned with health identity anyway as it is often blind to the healthy side of the prominent distinction sick/healthy. In exaggerating Luhmann's proposition, Simon (1999) even argues that the medical system operates with the functional code sick/non-sick, for the side of health leads to obscurity. However, health system(s) have a greater concern for health. Public health and health promotion systems would, in fact, impose and accentuate individual responsibility for one's health. These speculations bring us back to the idea of doing health identity in experiences of dentine sensitivity. The positive practices, where health responsibilities are taken up by individuals, transform into proactive management of the condition. Apart from adaptive management it could also involve proactive management and it was here that toothpaste emerged as a particular lifestyle choice.

Toothpaste as solution: help/cure and (positive) difference/change

A significant proportion of the interviewees (as much as the general population with sensitivity in teeth) have been active consumers of sensitive toothpastes. Sensitive toothpastes and other oral health products for sensitive teeth were launched onto the market in the 1980s, with Sensodyne being among the first brands. Today, pharmaceutical developments enable a wider population to make their own decisions on the choice of the product and particular brand. The positive effects of sensitive toothpaste on dentine caused the most exciting dilemmas: to date no one could be certain whether the toothpaste had to be qualified as a medicinal product such as OTC (or direct to consumer drug) or an oral hygiene (cosmetic) product with a health impact. Indeed one interviewee picked up and expanded on this dilemma of oral care: 'I see it more as prevention than a cure' (S2.3). By looking at the range of first-order forms prevention/cure, use/help, toothpaste/medicine and treatment/cure one could observe the importance of the distinction. Eventually, the second-order form help/cure resolved itself into a complex paradox:

> It's quite a lot of money, but it's some sort of, I'm not going to talk about everlasting treatment … you can't just get rid of something, you can't just cure something. It takes a lot longer but maybe just chewing gum, with Arginine in it, maybe some sort of everyday food, that as you eat it helps.
> (S2.2)

The form, therefore, suggested that toothpaste can't cure the sensitivity in teeth. No ultimate, everlasting treatment was feasible. Despite the fact that it is a 'short/sharp pain' its recurrence could stretch off into the future. Yet, using sensitive toothpaste helped. The product was 'working its magic' for the majority of users interviewed, and many embraced the idea of looking after themselves. At the same time there was an awareness that its treatment effects worked on an everyday basis. Some were saying that the resistance was building up slowly with constant application. In other words, the sensitive toothpaste seemed to provide a stable, consistent and comfortable strategy to be chosen proactively by people with sensitivity episodes. Using it, but also shopping for it, became a part of their oral care and health practices. On a larger scale, the paradox help/cure related the paradoxes of treatment-seeking behaviour, recognisable in other health conditions, where people strive for cure. Having said that, new promises of instant relief in recent pharmaceutical ads (Colgate) could potentially change the treatment-seeking paradox. Future studies will show.

Because the sensitive toothpaste had a positive effect for most of the individuals interviewed, the final set of forms pointed to the paradox of difference. Positive difference was noticed by many users, however, in various degrees; some admitted that the use of the specialised toothpaste 'was doing something', others confessed that it dismissed the sensitivity in teeth for them so that 'problem's 99 per cent solved'. A range of first-order forms lent some support to the solution: better/improvement, difference/stops, different/effective. Difference was negative too – once they have been deprived from the sensitive toothpaste (on a holiday, a trip, etc.): out of the toothpaste/difference. In interviews of this kind the participants shared that the sensitivity was back within two to three days. The paradox of difference involved the response to the change in both ways: in the case of resorting to the toothpaste and abstaining from it. All in all the experience of toothpaste was rewarding.

The second-order form (positive) difference/change emerged as the most reflective distinction in one particular interview:

> Probably it is a problem and I should do something about it so making the difference of buying the toothpaste and using that has made me realise that, hang on a second, I think there was something more to this and I probably was not right to live with it. I wasn't right, I should have probably tried to change it earlier.
>
> (2.14)

This quote disclosed another (the third) meaning of change – the difference that one can make by reinforcing one's own practices of oral health by consciously purchasing and applying the toothpaste on a daily basis. Indeed, for the toothpaste to be working a proactive consumer choice should be made, yet, the habits changing were the greatest behavioural change and challenge. 'I probably was not right to live with it' – addressed important questions of the self-management of dentine hypersensitivity. So far, leaving aside the complexity around consumer choices, our discussion centred on two crucial paradoxes, pertinent to toothpaste use: the treatment-seeking paradox and the paradox of difference. The toothpaste has been provided as a functional and indeed symbolic solution to the problem of dentine sensitivity. It may be said that it represents a pharmaceutical solution to the problem that constitutes one of the symbiotic mechanisms of the health system suggested by Pelikan (2007).

Conclusions

Luhmann's social systems theory offers a whole series of analytical techniques to understand the relationship between society and health. We hope that in this brief chapter we have been able to illustrate that his work can be used beyond the analysis of systems, system semantics and social differentiation amongst other things. His approach can in fact open up a new way for us to understand how health is communicated and in particular what it means for health systems when patients speak about their condition. We would just like to make a few small points here to indicate the significance of what is being discussed in this analysis.

The form analysis presented here, prompted by Luhmann's thinking, suggests a new way to understand and analyse interview data. It illuminates an alternative description of narratives of health by opening up the phenomena of distinctions. Searching for words with condensed meaning enabled us to explore a health condition such as dentine hypersensitivity with a unique perspective. Form analysis helped to shape the concise picture – sharp and short pain in teeth that individuals habitually try to minimise by retreating to self-deprivation and endurance or by the proactive use of sensitive toothpaste. Form analysis elegantly locks the logic of the interviewees into their own and very reflexive forms. It also demonstrates how complex forms could be paradoxical in their two sides: they played like a coin; each side was possible only if the other existed.

Our analysis disclosed six paradoxes of dentine hypersensitivity: the paradox of pain, the paradox of deprivation, the paradox of endurance, a paradox of health identity, the treatment-seeking paradox and the paradox of difference. As far as this particular oral condition was concerned we did not exhaust the list of forms. From our analysis there are several interesting implications. Both people and social systems share the medium of meaning, but in fact it might be possible that three of the forms mentioned here may have been treated by the health system as media. In particular we noted that the short/sharp distinction has in fact been copied into the scientific description of dentine sensitivity. If this is the case, and further analysis is needed to confirm this, this has significant implications for the importance of reporting signs and symptoms in health settings. The everyday communication of bodily symptoms might in fact be another very important symbolically generalisable media for health systems that could be set alongside Pelikan's (2007) differential diagnosis. We can go further than this however. We can suggest that the form of care/cure and the paradox of difference produce a distinctive pattern of response to dentine sensitivity. One accepts that the condition is always going to be present: it cannot be cured, but it can nonetheless be prevented by caring for it. Likewise we can see that the paradox of difference is an important form of evaluation for the solutions people use, in this case a desensitising technology: in the form of toothpaste. In this respect then the technology may have been able to draw on these forms to symbolically attach itself as the solution. Once more the health system may have been operating to utilise the forms communicated in the everyday experience of dentine sensitivity as its media. In short the technology communicates itself through these forms. We cannot be completely sure on this final point because to establish this requires further research into the historical semantics of some of these forms. These issues remain the subject of further analysis.

Note

1 For quite some time getting to grips with Luhmann's theory has been difficult. There are however, several very good introductions to the ideas in Luhmann's work in English. Two books in particular are highly recommended. There is the work of Hans-Georg Moeller (2006) *Luhmann Explained: From Souls to Systems* and the work of Michael King (2009) in *Systems, Not People, Make Society Happen*. Both books are quite different. Moeller's (2006) work seeks to provide an introduction to Luhmann by taking the reader through his way of thinking about society and then drawing on Luhmann's ideas on the mass media as a particular example of the empirical application of Luhmann's theory. The book is particularly useful for its careful referencing and in particular an extensive though not exhaustive bibliography of works from Luhmann and on Luhmann in English. It is a perfect place to start with the context of Luhmann's writing. King (2009) takes a completely different approach. His book is clearly set out to introduce the ideas of Luhmann from the perspective of his anti-humanism and seeks to avoid all contextualising debates. Both books are immensely helpful in clarifying Luhmann's ideas and should be read by anyone interested in contemporary social theory. Another text which is a 'must read' for those interested in developing applications of Luhmann's work is Niels Åkerstrom Andersen's (2003) excellent text *Discursive Analytical Strategies: Understanding Foucault, Koselleck, Laclau, Luhmann*.

In addition to these there are many other places where one can get a brief introduction to Luhmann, but like everything to do with any theoretical author there are probably as many interpretations of Luhmann as there are authors. One good example of a particular take on Luhmann is the work of John Mingers (Mingers, 2002, 1995) who introduces and critiques Luhmann's use of the concept of autopoiesis. Some of this work was later criticised by King and Thornhill (King and Thornhill, 2008) for misconstruing aspects of Luhamnn's systems theory. This is of course not to say that one could not innovate with Luhmann's approach; on the contrary, there are many excellent examples of work that has been inspired by Luhmann (Baecker, 1999, Rasch, 2000, Rasch and Wolfe, 2000, Qvortrup, 2003). On top of these books, each of which has a particular interest in Luhmann, there are a whole series of articles one can turn to which seek to provide an introduction to his ideas (Arnoldi, 2001, Baecker, 2001, Baecker, 2002). Despite all of these various introductions there remains very little on health from the perspective of Luhmann.

References

Andersen, N. A. 2003. *Discrusive analytical strategies: Understanding Foucault, Laclau and Luhmann*, Bristol: Policy Press.
Arato, A. 1994. Civil society and political theory in the work of Luhmann and beyond. *New German Critique*, 61, 129–42.
Armstrong D., Lilford R., Ogden J., Wessely S., 2007. Health-related quality of life and the transformation of symptoms. *Sociology of Health & Illness*, 29, 570–83.
Arnoldi, J. 2001. Niklas Luhmann: An Introduction. *Theory, Culture and Society*, 18, 1–13.
Baecker, D. 2001. Gypsy Reason: Niklas Luhmann's Sociological Enlightenment. *Cybernetics and Human Knowing*, 6, 5–19.
——2002. Why systems? *Theory, Culture and Society*, 18, 59–74.
——(ed.) 1999. *Problems of form*, Stanford, CA: Stanford University Press.

Bauch, J. 1996. *Gesundheit als sozialer Code. Von der Vergesellschaftung des Gesundheitswesens zur Medikalisierung der Gesellschaft*, Munchen: Juventa.
——2000. *Medizinsoziologie*, Munchen, Oldenburg.
Birenbaum-Carmeli, D. 2004. 'Cheaper than a newcomer': on the social production of IVF policy in Israel. *Sociology of Health & Illness*, 26, 897–924.
Boiko, O. V., Baker, S. R., Gibson, B. J., Locker, D., Sufi, F., Barlow, A. & Robinson PG., 2010. Construction and validation of the quality of life measure for dentine hypersensitivity (DHEQ). *Journal of Clinical Periodontology*, 37, 973–80.
Boiko, O. V., Ward, P., Robinson, P. G. and Gibson, B. J. 2011. Form and semantic of communication in dental encounters: oral health, probability and time. *Sociology of Health & Illness*, 33, (1), 16–32.
Canadian Advisory Board on Dentin Hypersensitivity. 2003. Consensus-Based Recommendations for the Diagnosis and Management of Dentin Hypersensitivity. *Journal of the Candian Dental Association*, 69, 221–26.
Dababneh, R., Khouri, A. T. and Addy, M. 1999. Dentine hypersensitivity – an enigma? A review of terminology, epidemiology, mechanisms, aetiology and management. *British Dental Journal*, 187, 606–11.
Fox, N. & Ward, K. 2006. Health identities: from expert patient to resisting consumer. *Health: An Interdisciplinary Journal for the Social Study of Health, Illness and Medicine*, 10, 461–479.
Gibson, B., Acquah, S. & Robinson, P. 2005. Recovering drug users and oral health: A Secondary Analysis of Qualitative Data. *British Dental Journal*, 198, 219–224.
Gibson, B., Boiko, O. V., Baker, S. R., Robinson, P., Barlow, A., Player T. and Locker, D. 2010. The everyday impact of dentine sensitivity: personal and functional aspects. *Social Science and Dentistry*, 1, 11–20.
Gilson, L. 2003. Trust and the development of health care as a social institution. *Social Science & Medicine*, 56, 1453–1468.
Gregory, J., Gibson, B. & Robinson, P. 2005. Variation and change in the meaning of oral health related quality of life: a 'grounded' systems approach. *Social Science & Medicine*, 60, 1859–1868.
Glotzer, D. E., Freedberg, K. A. and Bauchner, H. 1995. Management of Childhood Lead-Poisoning – Clinical Impact and Cost-Effectiveness. *Medical Decision Making*, 15, 13–24.
Harris, R. and Curtin, J. H. 1976. Dentine hypersensitivity. *Aust Dent J*, 21, 165–69.
Hornung, B. R. 2006. Luhmann's Legal and Political Sociology. In: King, M. and Thornhill, C. (eds.) *Luhmann on Law and Politics*. Oxford: Hart Publishing.
King, M. 2009. *Systems, not people, make Society Happen*, Holcombe Publishing.
King, M. and Thornhill, C. 2006. *Luhmann on law and politics: Critical Appraisals and applications*, Oxford: Hart Publishing.
——2003. *Niklas Luhmann's Theory of Politics*, New York, Palgrave Macmillan.
——2008. 'Will the real Niklas Luhmann stand up, please'. A reply to John Mingers. *The Sociological Review*, 51, 276–85.
Lonardi, C. 2007. The passing dilemma in socially invisible diseases: Narratives on chronic headache. *Social Science & Medicine*, 65, 1619–29.
Luhmann, N. 1983a. Anspruchsinflation im Krankheitssystem. Eine Stellungnahme aus gesellschaftstheoretischer Sicht. In: Herder-Dorneich, P. and Schuller, A. (eds.) *Die Anspruchsspirale: Schicksal oder Systemdefekt? 3. Kolle=ner Kolloquium*. Stuttgart: Kohlhammer.
——1983b. Medizin und Gesellschaftstheorie. *Medizin Mensch Gesellschaft*, 8, 168–75.
——1989. *Ecological Communication*, Cambridge: Polity Press.

———1990a. Der Medizinische Code. In: Luhmann, N. (ed.) *Soziologische Aufklarung 5. Konstruktivistische Perspektiven*. Opladen: Westdeutscher Verlag.
———1990b. The Paradox of System Differentiation and the Evolution of Society. In: Alexander, J. C. and Colomy, P. (eds.) *Differentiation Theory and Social Change: Comparative and Historical Perspectives*. New York: Columbia University Press.
———1991. *Political Theory in the Welfare State*, Berlin: Walter de Gruyter.
———1993. *Risk: A Sociological Theory*, New York: Aldine De Gruyter.
———1995. *Social Systems*, Stanford, CA: Stanford University Press.
———1998. *Observations on Modernity*, Stanford, CA: Stanford University Press.
———2002. *Theories of Distinction: Redescribing the Descriptions of Modernity*, Stanford, CA: Stanford University Press.
Luhmann, N. and Behnke, K. 1994. Speaking and Silence. *New German Critique*, 25–37.
Maturana, H. and Varela, F. 1980. Autopoiesis and Cognition: the Realization of the Living. In: Cohen, R. and Wartofsky, M. (eds.) *Boston Studies in the Philosophy of Science*. Boston, MA: Reidel Publishing Co.
Melzack, R. 1973. *The puzzle of pain*, Middlesex: Penguin Books.
Meyer, S., Ward, P., Coveney, J. & Rogers, W. 2008. Trust in the health system: An analysis and extension of the social theories of Giddens and Luhmann. *Health Sociology Review*, 17, 177–186.
Michailakis, D. & Schirmer, W. 2010. Agents of their health? How the Swedish welfare state introduces expectations of individual responsibility. *Sociology of Health & Illness*, 32, 930–947.
Mingers, J. 1995. *Self-Producing Systems: Implications and Applications of Autopoiesis*, New York: Plenum Press.
———2002. Can Social Systems be autopoietic? Assessing Luhmann's social theory. *The Sociological Review*, 50, 278–99.
Moeller, H.-G. 2006. *Luhmann Explained: From Souls to Systems*, Peru, Illinois, Open Court.
Murphy, J. W. and Pilotta, J. J. 1987. Research note: Identifying 'at risk' persons in community based research. *Sociology of Health & Illness*, 9, 62–75.
Osborne, T. 1993. James Mackenzie, General Practitioner: a modest contribution to the archaeology of clinical reason. *Sociology of Health and Illness*, 15, 525–46.
Pelikan, J. 2007. Understanding differentiation of Health in Late Modernity by use of Sociological Systems Theory. In: McQueen, D., Kickbusch, I., Potvin, L., Pelikan, J., Balbo, L. and Abel, T. (eds.) *Health and Modernity: The Role of Theory in Health Promotion*. New York: Springer Science.
Qvortrup, L. 2003. *The Hypercomplex Society*, Oxford: Peter Lang.
Rasch, W. 2000. *Niklas Luhmann's Modernity: The paradoxes of Differentiation*, Standford, CA: Stanford University Press.
Rasch, W. and Wolfe, C. 2000. *Observing Complexity: Systems Theory and Postmodernity*, Minneapolis: University of Minnesota Press.
Reznik, D. L., Murphy, J. W. and Belgrave, L. L. 2007. Globalisation and medicine in Trinidad. *Sociology of Health & Illness*, 29, 536–50.
Simon, F. B., 1999. The Other Side of Illness. In Baecker, D., 1999. *Problems of Form*. Stanford University Press, Stanford CA.
Spencer-Brown, G. 1969. *Laws of Form*, London: George Allen and Unwin.

5 Bourdieu and the impact of health and illness in the lifeworld

Sasha Scambler

Introduction

The premise upon which the work of Pierre Bourdieu (1990a; 1999; Bourdieu & Wacquant, 1992) is built is that the social world is not a naturally occurring phenomenon that can be understood through 'common sense' groupings or models such as that of family or culture. The phenomena that make up the social world in which we live are culturally and historically bounded and temporal in nature. Furthermore, they are socially constructed within a structural network of social and power relations (Jenkins 2002). Bourdieu's concepts of field and habitus seek to address the ways in which agency and reflexivity (habitus) are shaped by or embedded within structure (field). The framework he outlines offers a novel way of thinking about the complexities of the everyday experiences of life, incorporating structure and agency and providing a way of categorising the different forms of currency or capital that we use to negotiate the lifeworld and our place within it.

Whilst often categorised as a social theorist, Bourdieu claims his work is a means of interpreting the empirical world in which we live and rejects the notion of creating theory divorced from empirical enquiry. Jenkins explains Bourdieu's 'reluctance to theorise other than through a research based engagement with the complexities of social life' (2002: 176). Furthermore, he notes that the results of research into the social world produce an account of reality that is not 'reality' per se and is merely a product of the ways in which the account has been constructed, thus forcing the researcher and reader into a position of reflexivity. These are just some of the reasons why the theoretical framework outlined by Bourdieu has such potential within medical sociology in helping to explore and explain the complexities of living with illness, and particularly long-term illness or disability, and in forcing us to think about both the structure/agency debate and the role of the researcher.

This chapter starts then with an outline of Bourdieu's concepts of field, capital and habitus before providing a critical exposition of the Bourdieuian take on the structure/agency debate. It concludes with an example of how this framework could be used to rethink empirical data within the field of medical sociology.

Field and capital

The field can be defined as a social arena or space, bounded in an experiential context, in which actors attend to the self and/or a given situation. Fields are generated in any circumstances where practices are performed. They have within them a series of structural configurations, power and social relations, which influence the actions of all those who enter a given field and prompt certain types of behaviour, influenced by the distribution and transaction of various forms of capital, which may be field specific or cut across multiple fields. In the words of Bourdieu and Wacquant:

> [A] field may be defined as a network, or a configuration, of objective relations between positions. These positions are objectively defined, in their existence and in the determinations they impose on their occupants, agents and institutions, by their present and potential situation in the structure of the distribution of the species of power (or capital) whose possession commands access to the specific profits that are at stake in the field, as well as their objective relations to other positions ...
>
> (1992: 94)

Thus the field can be seen as a structured space in which people act, and which is both shaped by the actions of those within it and imposes constraints on those actions, and capital is the resource used to negotiate through and act within the field. Capital may be transferred between fields, but is 'context-specific' and so may hold different values in different fields (Behague et al. 2008). Thus, capital must be transformed to fit into each new field and may, in the process, gain or lose value. 'Fields, then, are the sites for power-struggles over capital and over the determination of legitimate and illegitimate actions of that field' (ibid.: 492).

Four specific forms of capital are identified by Bourdieu. These are economic, social, cultural and symbolic capital, and they operate throughout and across fields. Economic capital is directly convertible to commodity forms such as money and is institutionalised through laws such as those concerning property rights. Within the fields of disease and disability for example, economic capital may be used to refer to the money available to adapt to and combat a disease, through personal wealth, income, benefits and state intervention. This economic capital is institutionalised through the health and welfare systems and through legislation on work and pay conditions. Cultural capital is based on socially 'legitimated' knowledge and practices, which in certain circumstances is convertible to economic capital and is institutionalised through educational qualifications and membership of professional bodies. In a health context, the accumulation and ability to mobilize this form of capital is relevant to debates around the legitimated power of the medical profession or the professionalisation of allied groups such as dentists or nurses. Social capital is linked to relations with others, incorporating affiliations and social obligations as well as familial, friendship and other networks. Social capital may also be convertible to economic capital and is institutionalised through social networks. This type of capital can be found in the formal and informal support networks available to people living with a broad range of conditions, diseases, disabilities or experiences, as represented by the proliferation of virtual self-help groups and forums that have emerged over the past decade.

The final type of capital Bourdieu identifies is symbolic capital. This relates to the prestige, status and honour ascribed to significant institutions, groups and social relations that, in certain circumstances, are convertible to economic capital. This form of capital is institutionalised through systems that ascribe status such as the peerage system or that associated with parental authority, or seniority within a tribe or family. Interesting dynamics occur in the health field, for example when the symbolic capital of individual adults or parents are challenged by, or clash with, health policy or the legitimated cultural capital of the medical profession. This can create barriers to the mobilization of capital for people within the field. To these four forms of capital, Williams (1995) suggests that we add the concept of physical capital when using a Bourdieuian framework within medical sociology. Physical capital, he suggests, relates to the health, fitness for purpose and aesthetic quality of the body through which actors embody habitus within the field. As we shall see later, this idea of physical capital is partly captured with Bourdieu's use of the concept of bodily hexis (1977) to refer to the manner and style in which actors carry themselves. For Bourdieu, this is the point at which the personal (habitus) and the social (field and capital) combine. In the context of sociological work in the field of health and illness, however, it may indeed be useful to think of the health-related, aesthetic and functional qualities of the body as capital that can be mobilized and transacted with as actors negotiate their way through the field.

The nature of the field and the structure within it determines the configuration of forces within the field, and the inter and intra balances of power within and between species of capital and fields. Although the accrual of capital yields power, capital requires a field in which to operate. As such, primary aims of agents in the field are maintaining and improving (or preventing devaluation) of their position. Similarly, cultural commonalities, repeated social hierarchies and even patterns of bodily form and deportment are reproduced through practice, and evaluated and accorded differential status and social, cultural and economic values in a pre-existing field according to the structures at work within that field. In a health context, therefore, McDonnell et al. (2009) suggest that the capacity individuals have to accumulate and transact with capital in ways that are beneficial to health are dependent to a large extent on the wider structural impact of inequalities. If social capital, for example, is 'linked to possession of a durable network of more or less institutionalised relationships of mutual acquaintance and recognition' (Bourdieu 1986: 248), the accumulation and mobilisation of this for capital is, therefore, dependent on social power, which, in turn, is determined by wider socio-economic structures. The social networks that Bourdieu alludes to can 'work exclusively by giving group members access to influence and material resources' (McDonnell et al. 2009: 20). Social capital, along with economic, cultural and symbolic capital, can thus be seen as intrinsically linked with the dynamics of class formation, structuring the ability of individuals to exercise choice. Whilst people have choice over whether or not they behave in ways that may be detrimental to their health, these choices are constrained by the social context in which the choices are made and the structural dynamics within that context. The role of agency, choice and individual action is the concern of the second part of Bourdieu's theoretical framework, and his concept of habitus.

Habitus

Habitus is the agentic aspect of Bourdieu's theory and reflects the unthinking or unconscious ways in which people act on a day-to-day basis. These actions are shaped by the knowledge that we acquire through the process of socialisation (Layder 1994) and by the social context or field in which habitus is exercised. Habitus, thus, is 'a socially influenced disposition to think or act in particular ways.' (McDonnell *et al.* 2009: 43). When seen in the context of health, the ways in which our bodies act 'become shaped through daily unconscious practices that are nonetheless related to social relations of class, gender and ethnicity operating in society' (ibid.: 43). Thus, whilst people have choices over their adoption of health behaviours that promote or are detrimental to health, these choices are linked to the material and cultural constraints of the social milieu in which people live and thus are constrained or bounded choices (McDonnell *et al.* 2009).

Habitus, therefore, according to Bourdieu, consists of a set of embodied dispositions, the parameters of which are set through the context or field, which shape behaviour and personal/social expectations. Thus, through the interaction between field, habitus and capital, action can be said to produce and reproduce structure. Structure exists through constructive practices (Adams 2006). Actors move through a variety of fields in our daily lives but tend, Bourdieu suggests, to move within fields that are common to our social groupings. As such we develop an unconscious or tacit understanding of how to act in these fields. Bourdieu (1990) refers to this as 'doxic' experience, whereby internal and external structures are mutually constitutive resulting in unconscious practices. We 'have a feel for the game' and a knowledge of how to act in a given field. This is not, however, to suggest that all action is unconscious, and the term 'doxic habitus' is utilised to refer to deliberate or intentional actions that nevertheless emerge through, or are located within, the logic of experiences of reality within a known social context. In his own words: 'Each agent, wittingly or unwittingly, willy nilly, is producer and reproducer of objective meaning ... it is because the subjects do not, strictly speaking, know what they are doing that what they do has more meaning than they know' (cited in Williams 1995: 582). Structurally positioned effects can thus be said to precede or at the very least coexist alongside autonomous action. Thus, ' ... people's wills adjust to their possibilities' because 'they have a taste for what they are anyway condemned to' (Bourdieu 1990: 216; Bourdieu cited in Williams 1995: 594).

It is clear from this that, whilst there is space for individual choice and conscious actions, these are shaped by structural factors.

[W]hat Bourdieu described are subconscious culturally determined templates or dispositions which inform behaviour and importantly generate different forms of capital for an individual in different settings (…). He also typologised these cultural templates on the basis of class and argued that the characteristics of those templates inform and reinforce inter-class power relations together with facets such as health behaviour. When a person's habitus and field are congruent they develop important social, economic and psychological capital that provide the resources of life. If, however, something interferes with that congruence their capacity to develop such capital is compromised.'

(Forbes and Wainwright 2001: 806)

Thus our capacity to accumulate and transact with capital is mitigated by the degree of congruity between habitus and field. Again this has interesting implications for the study of people living with long-term, profoundly disabling conditions where they may find themselves in a non-doxic field where they do not know how to act, they do not have the 'feel for the game'. Not only does this affect their actions within the field but it also inhibits their ability to accumulate and transact with the capital needed to successfully negotiate the field in which they find themselves. An example of how Bourdieu's theory can be used to explore the experiences of people who find themselves in non-doxic fields through the diagnosis of a long-term, profoundly disabling condition is given in the final part of the chapter.

Awareness of moving through a non-doxic field and the need to adapt and moderate habitus within the field is referred to by Bourdieu as reflexivity. An individual's capacity for reflexive thought may develop as an altered form of habitus or as a required constituent of a particular field. Bourdieu uses the example of academia as a field where reflexivity is actively encouraged, in his epistemological critique of social research – and in particular the key notions of 'participant objectification' and the 'objectification of objectification' – he suggests that the reflexivity of the researcher is central to social research (Jenkins 2002). It is also important to note that reflexivity is exercised within a structured environment. Thus the parent who seeks to develop medical knowledge and skills to enable them to best care for a child with a rare condition must fight to get their knowledge and skills legitimated within the dominant biomedical structure in which they find themselves (Scambler and Newton 2011). Similarly, parents seeking to transmit dominant cultural values through involvement in their children's education may face a greater challenge if the field of academia is non-doxic (Reay, 1998). Thus 'middle class women are predominantly engaging in a process of replicating habitus while their working class counterparts are attempting a much harder task; that of transforming habitus'. In this way 'choices' given to people, whether concerning the type of school that their children attend, or the hospital which best meets their particular needs, may be rendered meaningless to those who lack the resources to make a meaningful choice. This has a particular resonance if one considers the changes to the National Health Service orchestrated by the Conservative and Liberal Democrat Coalition government, which trumpet the centrality of 'choice'.

In the field of health, habitus has been characterised as one of passivity and compliance. The power structure of the field within which health habitus is enacted is one in which medical and allied professionals take the position of power and control the interactions. In their work on the use of medication in old age, Lumme-Sandt and Virtanen (2002) showed that, whilst the default habitus is passive and compliant, many patients actively used capital accumulated within other fields, particularly employment, to negotiate and change health habitus. Similarly, Angus *et al.* (2005) suggest that biographical and biological crises, such as those that are represented in the chronic illness literature (see Bury 1982), may lead to changes in both habitus and social position. The role of capital and habitus is explored in Behague *et al.*'s work (2008) in which they used Bourdieu's theoretical framework to explore the negotiation of blame and responsibility in the context of severe or near-death obstetric events. In their study of 74 women who experienced severe obstetric events, only one-third made a complaint despite evidence of widespread poor practice. Examination of the role of patient feedback in changing quality of care suggested that a lack of capital resources combined with low status in the hierarchy of the field itself (lack of power, low socio-economic status, being female) made patients reluctant to criticise healthcare practices even in the face of poor practice. Thus the passivity is structural. For these women, low status in the health field was often combined with negotiation of a range of complex social fields, with problematic marriages, family networks and a lack of material resources. This resulted in women with low health habitus being assigned and accepting blame and responsibility for the event, even where care was of poor quality. In contrast, the minority of women who were able to complain had strong social support and advocates who were able to reinforce the patient. This resulted in traumatic events becoming catalysts for improving care rather than increasing the estrangement of the patient.

Habitus and bodily hexis

Not only is habitus agentic, it is also an embodied concept for Bourdieu. Habitus only exists in so much as it is in the heads of those who act. It exists in, through and because of the actions of the actors and is apparent in ways of moving, talking and using the body. Habitus, therefore, is not abstract. Neither is it simply manifest in behaviour; it is an integral part of embodied behaviours. Bourdieu suggests further that people act through an understanding of practical taxonomies that give order to actions. These include an understanding of male/female, front/back, hot/cold, up/down. Again he stresses that these practical taxonomies are rooted in the body, they are determined by the senses. The embodied nature of habitus is referred to by Bourdieu as bodily hexis. Bodily hexis is the manner and style in which actors carry themselves and is where the personal combines with the social. It is also where illness, disability or bodily abnormality affects the actors and may become visible or obvious.

From a sociological perspective, bodily hexis or the embodied nature of habitus is a useful tool for exploring the impact of illness and disability on everyday life.

Bodily hexis can be fundamentally affected by chronic or long-term conditions or by disability. Jenkins describes bodily hexis as

> a political mythology realised, embodied, turned into a permanent disposition, a durable manner of standing, speaking and thereby of feeling and thinking ... the principles embodied in this way are placed beyond the grasp of consciousness, and hence cannot be touched by voluntary, deliberate transformation, cannot even be made explicit ... for Bourdieu the body is a mnemonic device upon or in which the very basics of the habitus are emprinted in a socialising or learning process which commences during early childhood'.
>
> (2002: 75–76)

If bodily hexis is unknowable or beyond consciousness as it emerges from our social upbringing this raises the question as to what happens to unconscious bodily hexis when the body is impaired. Does the body's inability to be socialised raise bodily hexis into consciousness? This raises further questions about whether a new altered form of bodily hexis emerges or whether an impaired bodily hexis emerges. And what is the impact of this on habitus and the accumulation and transaction of capital? This has the potential to give us a new understanding of disability and potentially a way to develop a new theory that incorporates both the structural facets of disability theory encapsulated in oppression, and the experiential facets of the sociology of chronic illness and disability encapsulated in stigma and coping.

The structure/agency debate

In his 1990b work, 'In Other Words', Bourdieu refers to his work as 'genetic structuralism'. Jenkins describes his place in the structure agency debate as:

> ... the attempt to understand how 'objective', supra-individual social reality (cultural and institutional social structure) and the internalised 'subjective' mental worlds of individuals as cultural beings and social actors are inextricably bound up together, each being a contributor to – and, indeed, an aspect of – the other.
>
> (2002: 19–20)

In his book *The Logic of Practice* (1990a) Bourdieu attempts to transcend the choice between subjectivism and objectivism. Drawing on the work of Marx, he suggests that all social life is essentially practical, and that practice is located in space and time. Practice can be observed, therefore, in three dimensions and is defined by its place in time. Time, he suggests, in our understanding of it, is socially constructed. It is, however, socially constructed out of natural cycles – day and night, seasons and so forth (Jenkins 2002). If this is accepted, then social phenomena cannot be understood outside of time and space and any analysis of practice must, therefore, treat temporality as a central feature of its very nature. Bourdieu goes on to suggest that practice is not wholly orchestrated consciously, but nor does it just happen. We have what he calls a 'feel for the game', 'the practical mastery of the logic or of the imminent necessity of a game – mastery acquired by experience of the game, and one that works outside conscious control and discourse' (Jenkins, 2002: 70). Again, this links to Marx's idea that men make their own history but do not do so in circumstances of their own choosing (cited in Jenkins 2002: 70).

We have already established that we are socialised into a way of acting that is largely, although not wholly, unconscious, and that our body acts in ways appropriate or resonant with our habitus in a similarly unconscious manner. In addition, we grow up learning a set of practical cultural competencies, including a social identity or a sense of the position that we occupy in space. If you accept these arguments, this makes it very difficult to perceive social reality as anything other than the way things are, necessary to our own experience of who we are. Jenkins (2002) suggests that most people, most of the time, take themselves and their social world somewhat for granted. They do not think about it because they do not have to. This is doxic experience. Structure is portrayed by Bourdieu as an uneven set of positions within a power structure, which are defined by the spread and accumulation of various forms of capital and which produce or help to shape a particular type of habitus. Williams (1995) sees this as a way of explaining how 'subjective expectations' are aligned with 'objective probabilities'. Again the implications for health policy – which focuses on choice and behaviour change as keys to the emancipation of socio-economically disadvantaged people into a life of health – are not taking into account the structural limitations of choice and behaviour if viewed in this way.

Bourdieu's work also contains potential explanations for why expectations appear to match access to capital and resources. These he terms illusion and symbolic violence. Illusion relates to the internalisation of the doxic relationship whereby people have an understanding of the rules by which they are living and define themselves within the bounds of these rules (Newton 2009). Thus their expectations are shaped by their circumstances, albeit through thought rather than physically. In congruence, symbolic violence relates to the idea that the hierarchy and concomitant inequalities resultant from the unequal access to and distribution of capital are naturalised. This is similar to Marx's concept of false consciousness, whereby people internalise the dominant ideology without being aware that they do so. Wainwright (1996) suggests that this can lead to individualised or even pathological explanations for individual behaviours or even for inequalities themselves. Symbolic capital occurs at the point where different forms of capital collide and impact on the possibilities open to individuals, whether in relation to educational expectations and achievements or class-related definitions of health (Newton 2009). Williams (1995) takes this a step further to suggest that a Bourdieuian analysis can elucidate the structured nature of health concepts such as lifestyle, health behaviour and understandings of wellbeing and how these differentially structured concepts lead to differential behaviours, service utilisation and health outcomes. Furthermore, those at the top of the structural hierarchy within a field are in a position to determine the criteria through which judgements of taste and distinction are made. As Newton suggests: 'This, when combined with a notion of reflexivity as driven by contextual (field) mechanisms of propagation, explains the transmission of values and the mimetic embodiment of cultural forms and a structural determination of proclivity and its relation to uneven, class based outcomes' (2009: 123). It is only in a non-doxic field that the potential for non-habitus bound reflexivity becomes apparent in the conscious decisions that people make about how they need to act and the capital that they need to accumulate to negotiate themselves successfully through a non-doxic field.

Criticisms of Bourdieu's work range from his own criticism of his struggle to use language effectively to get across the points that he wishes to make (1988) to his perceived failure to overcome the objectivist/subjectivist divide within his work (Jenkins 2002). The main criticisms of Bourdieu's work stem from the charge that he is unnecessarily structurally deterministic (see Adams 2006) and, whilst talking about agency, has developed a concept of agency that is structurally bounded. Jenkins (2002) suggests that habitus can be seen as unconscious actions structured by power relations, social class and differentiated access to capital with little if any room for conscious thought, agency or choice. People think they are thinking about the world and making choices about how they live, but in fact they are only doing this within a set of predetermined options available to them. Further, Archer (2007) suggests that life is less structured than Bourdieu's reliance on socialisation suggests, and that we regularly encounter situations with which we are unfamiliar and have to think about how to act in these situations. Thompson (1991) goes as far as to state that in his quest to overcome the subjectivism/objectivism debate Bourdieu fails because he is unable to let go of his underlying belief that objectivism is 'less inadequate' than subjectivism, and thus comes down on the determinist side of the argument. There are also criticisms of Bourdieu's failure to clearly explain the nature of the concept of habitus or how it is related to that of culture (Jenkins 2002). If taken as a philosophy or a 'grand narrative', there are clearly contradictions and there is a lack of clarity in Bourdieu's work. This is not, however, how he intended his work to be used. As noted in the introduction, Bourdieu intended his work to be used as a means of exploring and seeking to explain empirical data rather than a social theory per se; his work gives us tools with which to think about the world. It is in this vein that the final part of the chapter illustrates one possible way in which Bourdieu's 'social theory' can be used to explore and explain empirical data.

Bourdieu in practice: an exploration of the field of Batten disease

The work of Bourdieu, as previously acknowledged, has been utilised to explore the implications of health, illness and disability by a number of researchers (see Williams 1995, Behague *et al.*, 2008, Ming-cheng and Stacey 2008, Huppatz 2009). One such study utilised Bourdieu's concepts of field, habitus and capital to explore the experiences of families of children with Batten disease on entering a non-doxic, biologically bounded field (Scambler and Newton 2010, 2011). Empirical data taken from qualitative interviews with the families of children with Batten disease were analysed, using a Bourdieuian framework, in an attempt to encapsulate the causal swamping of the lifeworld by the biological within the field of Batten disease whilst acknowledging both capital flows and individual agency.

Batten disease can be characterised as a biologically 'overwhelming', rare and chronically disabling, degenerative group of diseases (Siintola *et al.* 2006). The global prevalence of the group of diseases is thought to be approximately 1:12.500 (Hofmann and Peltonen 2001), although this is likely to be an underestimation owing to poor recording in many countries. When considered as a group, however, the prevalence of the lysosomal storage disorders as a whole is closer to 1:5000, giving the experiences of people living with diseases within this group considerably wider application. Batten disease is the common name for a group of rare, genetic, neurodegenerative, metabolic diseases that are found in both adults and children across the world. There are different types of Batten disease that are usually classified by age of onset into infantile (six months to two years); late infantile and variant late infantile (two to four years); juvenile (five to nine years); and an adult onset type. Age at onset, life expectancy, progress of symptoms and genetic causes vary by disease type; however, common symptoms include epilepsy, visual impairment, cognitive and motor degeneration (including the loss of the abilities to walk, eat and talk) and a shortened life expectancy (Scriver *et al.* 2001). At present there is no cure or treatment that makes a significant impact on the progressive decline in bodily functions and inevitable early death. Batten disease has a multifaceted and multilayered effect on the lifeworlds of all those it touches. This can be causally attributed to the biological attributes of the disease, but it is biological, social and psychological in its impact. The biological impact of the disease is both direct in its determination of the disease symptoms and the nature of the disease progression, and indirect in its impact on every, or almost every, aspect of daily life. Even the direct biological impact of the disease spreads far beyond the affected, diagnosed individual. The hereditary nature of Batten disease spreads the direct biological impact to siblings and extended family members and, potentially, to future generations through a network of carrier, post- and prenatal testing.

We have argued elsewhere (Scambler and Newton 2010) that unpicking the complex web of interrelated experiences, choices and actions that occur requires a theoretical framework that encapsulates both the bounded, and yet transient and permeable, nature of the field itself as well as the power relations and extant positions that occur within it. The work of Bourdieu can be used to encapsulate the causal swamping of the lifeworld by the biological within the field of Batten disease, while acknowledging both capital flows and the array of roles and positions available within this social arena. By envisaging Batten disease as a field with biologically determined parameters, we can explore the ways in which the disease and all it entails imposes on agents who find themselves within it. The parameters of the field are temporal and temporary in that they are dependent on the changing and developing realms of biological and biomedical research into both the genetic makeup and mechanisms of the disease itself, as well as the development of potential therapies for 'treatment' or care. We chart the changing nature of behaviour exhibited by families on entering the field, occurring at the point of symptom onset. Following this, relational configurations in the field are largely arranged through how capital flows can represent and correspond to the impact of the biological. The exit point of the field is pressingly temporal – the irreversible progression towards death. The field is entered through the formal process of diagnosis, in which affected children receive the requisite label and families receive the legitimation of their place within the field. Months or years of tests, indeterminate symptoms and misdiagnoses can lead to families lingering on the periphery of the field, sometimes for extended periods of time, while awaiting the legitimation required to enter the field and be formally recognised, and in the interim facing potential challenges to their right to even linger on the periphery. Parents find themselves in the position of fighting for entrance into a field to which they would rather not belong, but once entered, wish to remain in as long as possible. Further to this, inherent within a field is a structured system of social positions and power relations formed by the interplay and distribution of various species of capital, which may cut across multiple fields. These positions develop because of the fact that positions occupied within the field afford or deny access to the distribution of resources within a field. The parameters of the field are biological. The gatekeepers' influence is, thus, biomedical in nature, stemming from the utilisation and representation of the biological to generate and maintain power in accordance with existing modes of capital in wider society.

As already outlined, Bourdieu distinguishes four key forms or species of capital that operate throughout fields: economic, cultural, social and symbolic. In addition, we draw on Williams' (1995) concept of 'physical capital', which is of particular relevance to those existing within a field with biologically determined parameters. These five forms of capital are open to disruption, depletion and devaluation on entry into the field of Batten disease. To summarise:

> Economic capital in the field of Batten disease can refer to the money available to families to adapt to and combat the disease, through personal wealth, benefits and state intervention. This economic capital is institutionalised through the health and welfare systems, and wider social patterning through employment, taxation, entitlement and so on. Empirical evidence suggests that the disease process impacts upon the ability of parents of children with disabilities to accumulate economic capital while requiring increasing economic capital outlay.

Cultural capital may be challenged on entering the field of Batten disease as both existing cultural capital reserves and the ability to build more capital hinge on biomedical expertise. Moreover, previous cultural referrals and repertoires become devalued, devalorised or disjunctive in an arena where expert, specialised knowledge is seen to be the most appropriate wayfarer, and where parents must be able to respond on a day-to-day basis to the manifestations of the illness, as well as develop the ability to acquire new knowledge and practices around the disease process. In addition, as capital is determined largely in a biomedical capacity, parents are frequently ascribed contradictory and confusing positions in the circumstantial role array of the social arena – flitting, for example, from provider to parent to carer to proxy patient, and having to manage relations and concomitant institutional resources (usually) in the margins of each social network impacting on existing social capital.

Social capital refers to affiliations and obligations in relations pertaining to social obligations and quality of relations with others, which may also be convertible to economic capital, and is institutionalised through social networks. This type of capital can be found in the formal and informal support networks available to and drawn on by families, and may be challenged by the loss or non-repetition of previous forms of support.

Symbolic capital in the form of parental authority may be challenged by a multitude of professional experts with higher levels of biologically legitimated symbolic capital within the field of Batten disease. New avenues for collecting this type of capital are needed as parents develop and extend their parental authority into biomedical decision making, practice and potentially an altogether new status as an expert patient by proxy. This opens the door to a different, limited and field-specific form of capital, personal capital, into which, while allowing bounded entrance into the relations within the Batten disease field, these skills are predominantly non-transferable.

Physical capital is only relevant to the parents in this argument in so much as it holds up to the strain of providing care (seen in the effects of psychological morbidity as discussed earlier). We suggest that another relevant form of physical capital in this field is the loss or challenge to physical capital by proxy, by the impact of the disease process on the lives of the children and young adults living with Batten disease, that is, the sheer amount of physical, psychological and temporal impact, which is devoted to meet the everchanging ramifications and effects of the disease.

In Batten disease the configuration of forces within the field are positioned in relation to representing biology and responding to its impact – with professionals being positioned as legitimate delegates, holders and keepers of capital within the field. Thus, for families entering the field they must compete not just to accrue capital but to have their capital resources legitimated by those who hold dominant forms of capital within the field. Although the accrual of capital yields power, capital requires a field in which to operate. As such, primary aims of agents in the field are the maintenance and improvement of their position (or prevention of its devaluation). This may lead to a position where families fight to gain capital and legitimation for that capital, and professionals fight to prevent legitimation of types of capital that threaten their pre-existing positions and power within the field (for examples, see Baxter 1989, Case 2000). Parental capital stores can also be co-opted or bypassed by professionals claiming to represent the interests of the child as an 'individual'.

The final components of Bourdieu's framework in relation to our argument are habitus and reflexivity. Habitus relates to actions taken or responses to experiences within the field, and reflexivity is a process of seeking a context for the content of their experiences. Diagnosis puts some perspective on experiences to date, providing a brief sense of clarity, but the 'causal swamping' of biology leaves them with a certainty of more uncertainty rather than their previous (uninformed) uncertainty. Parents are also impelled to examine their existing habitus to find convergence, confluence, utility and room for adaptation in light of entry to the new field. This is particularly relevant here as we present a field that changes the social world in which families find themselves, and not only destroys, albeit temporarily, their capacity to produce capital but also assaults reserves built up in other more congruent fields. This can include the loss of reserves of social capital through the loss of friendship support networks, and the loss of economic and symbolic capital through the curtailment or cessation of careers and the status they ascribe. Thus, parents have to find a way of negotiating an unknown field with little knowledge about the resources that are needed or how they might accumulate them. Parents use the 'acquired knowledge' (Layder 1994) that they have brought into the field to shape the ways in which they respond, drawing on the capital that they have already accumulated while developing an understanding of the capital that they are going to need in order to 'act' effectively within the field, and of how that capital might be accrued. For those willing and able to exercise reflexivity, this process started at or before the point of diagnosis and would carry them throughout their visit to the field. It is in the negotiation that takes place around capital that the permeation of the biological becomes apparent in this field. The permeation of biology moves from the determination and policing of the parameters of the field itself, to, not only the control of their potential to act (having to respond to its effects and ramifications through care, knowledge, decision making and so forth), but control of the transactions that take place within the field (what is valid, valorised, available and so forth).

Using Bourdieu's theory in this way encapsulates the complexity of the experiences of these families at a structural, practical and emotional level and provides a framework through which the day–to-day experiences of the families can be understood and interpreted (for a more detailed analysis of this framework, illustrated with empirical data, see Scambler and Newton 2010, 2011).

Conclusions

Bourdieu describes his theory as a tool to help researchers to think about their empirical data, a practical framework through which individual experiences can be contextualised, incorporating individual action and structure in a way that allows us to explore both individual actions and choices and the structural factors that shape or influence these actions. In this chapter I make the case that Bourdieu's framework can offer us a sophisticated way of exploring the impact of health on daily life, whether through examining healthcare encounters (Behague *et al.* 2008), exploring the negotiation of health and medication (Lumme-Sandt and Virtanen 2002), or charting the daily lives of people living with long-term conditions (Scambler and Newton 2010, 2011). The ability to define a specific field, whether it be a medical condition, a healthcare setting or an overarching category such as health or disability, allows us to look at the boundaries of the field and the mechanisms through which people enter or leave the field, as well as the impact of the structures and power relations within that field in relation to the actions, experiences and daily lives of people within it. The possibility of focusing on one field without excluding the multiple other fields within which we act on a daily basis also enables us to look at the impact of the structure of a field on capital flows, accumulation and legitimation. This is of interest where, for example, the receipt of a diagnosis impacts on an individual's ability to accumulate or use capital, affecting daily life.

There is plenty of evidence that the types of capital outlined by Bourdieu are affected by health, illness, old age, social class, disability and many other areas of interest to medical sociologists. Disabled people earn less, on average, than their non-disabled peers, whilst some chronic conditions have been shown to affect social relations, family relations and the ability to hold down a job. Similarly there is plenty of evidence that social class affects health-care encounters. An exploration of capital flows within and across clearly defined fields allows us to contextualise the patterns that have been apparent in the literature for many years. This framework gives us the means to look at some old questions in a new way. What is the impact of living with a disability on capital accumulation, transaction and legitimation? How much of this impact is due to the personal, individual experience of the disability (demonstrated through pain, physical limitations or impairment); how much is through learned behaviour and the expectations of self and others (low self-esteem, communication difficulties, limited expectations); and how much is due to structural limitations inherent within the field? An analysis of the structure of the field and capital flows, along with habitus and bodily hexis, allows us to look at these questions not just individually or as a dichotomous relationship but symbiotically. How much of agency is shaped by structure? Bourdieu suggests that we may act in ways that we choose, but that our choices are largely shaped by socialisation. Thus we learn to make the choices that fit with our position in the field. This has major implications for people who find themselves in a non-doxic or unfamiliar field such as that defined by a long-term condition or a disability. If bodily hexis relates to learned and accepted ways of carrying ourselves, what are the implications for people performing bodily hexis with bodies that do not fit the norms, whether functionally or aesthetically? A multi-level analysis of this type has the potential to allow medical sociologists and disability theorists to work together, within the same framework, without losing the thrust of the disciplinary differences in approach. There are clearly limitations to Bourdieu's work if seen as a pure theory that seeks to elucidate the relationship between structure and agency. If, however, it is used as he intended, as a tool for the exploration of empirical data, there is huge potential for examining old arguments and debates in new ways.

References

Adams, M. (2006) Hybridizing Habitus and Reflexivity: Towards an Understanding of Contemporary Identity? *Sociology.* 40 (3): 511–28.

Angus J., Kontos, P., Dyck, L., McKeerer, P. & Poland, B. (2005) The personal significance of the home: habitus and the experience of receiving long term home care. *Sociology of Health and Illness.* 27 (2): 161–87.

Archer, M. S. (2007) *Making Our Way Through the World: Human Reflexivity and Social Mobility.* Cambridge: Cambridge University Press.

Baxter, C. (1989) Parent-perceived attitudes of professionals: Implications for service providers. *Disability, Handicap and Society.* 4 (3): 259–69.

Behague, D. P., Kanhonou, L. G., Filippi, V., Legonou, S. and Ronsmans, C. (2008) Pierre Bourdieu and transformative agency: a study of how patients in Benin negotiate blame and accountability in the context of severe obstetric events. *Sociology of Health and Illness.* 30 (4): 489–510.

Bourdieu, P. (1977) *Outline of a Theory of Practice.* Cambridge: Cambridge University Press.

——(1986) The Forms of Capital. In: *Handbook of Theory and Research for the Sociology of Education,* J. G. Richardson (ed.) Westport, CT: Greenwood Press.

——(1988) *Homo Academicus.* Translated by Peter Collier. Stanford, CA: Stanford University Press.

——(1990a) *The Logic of Practice.* Cambridge: Polity Press.

——(1990b) *In Other Words: Essays towards a Reflexive Sociology.* Cambridge: Polity Press.

——(1999) *The Weight of the World: Social Suffering in Contemporary Society.* Cambridge: Polity Press.

Bourdieu, P. and Wacquant, L. J. D. (1992) *An Invitation to Reflexive Sociology.* Cambridge: Polity Press.

Bury, M. (1982) Chronic Illness as Biographical Disruption. *Sociology of Health and Illness.* 4 (2): 167–82.

Case, S. (2000) Refocusing on the parent: Social issues for parents of disabled children. *Disability and Society.* 15 (2): 271–92.

Forbes, A. and Wainwright, S. (2001) On the Methodological, Theoretical and Philosophical context of Health Inequalities Research: A Critique. *Social Science & Medicine.* 53: 801–16.

Hofmann, S. L. and Peltonen, L. (2001) The Neuronal Ceroid Lipofuscinoses, In C. R. Scriver, A. L. Beaudet, W. S. Sly, B. Childs, B. Vogelstein (eds.) The Metabolic and Molecular Bases of Inherited Disease, 8th Edition. New York: McGraw-Hill.

Huppatz, K. (2009) Reworking Bourdieu's Capital: Feminine and Female Capitals in the Field of Paid Caring Work. *Sociology.* 43 (1): 45–66.

Jenkins, R. (2002) *Pierre Bourdieu.* Key Sociologists Series. Oxford: Routledge.

Layder, D. (1994) *Understanding Social Theory.* London: Sage.

Lumme-Sandt, K. and Virtanen, P. (2002) Older people in the field of medication. *Sociology of Health and Illness.* 24 (3): 285–304.

McDonnell, O., Lohan, M., Hyde, A. and Porter, S. (2009) *Social Theory, Health and Healthcare.* Cambridge: Palgrave MacMillan.

Ming-cheng, M. L. and Stacey, C. L. (2008) Beyond Cultural Competency: Bourdieu, patients and clinical encounters. *Sociology of Health and Illness.* 30 (5): 741–55.

Newton, P. D. (2009) The construction of selfhood as a social settlement in health: A qualitative study in Type 2 Diabetes. Unpublished PhD Thesis. King's College London.

Reay, D. (1998) Cultural Reproduction: Mothers' Involvement in Their Children's Primary Schooling. In: *Bourdieu and Education: Acts of Practical Theory*, M. Grenfell and D. James (eds) London: Routledge.

Scambler, S. and Newton, P. (2010) 'Where the Biological Predominates': Habitus, Reflexivity and Capital Accrual within the field of Batten Disease. In *New Directions in the Sociology of Chronic and Disabling Conditions: Assaults on the Lifeworld*, London: Routledge.

——(2011) Capital Transactions, Disruptions and the Emergence of Personal Capital in a Lifeworld Under Attack. *Social Theory and Health*. 9: 130–146.

Scriver, C. R., Beaudet, A. L., Sly, W. S., Childs, B. and Vogelstein, B. (eds.) (2001) *The Neuronal Ceroid Lipofuscinoses*. New York: McGraw-Hill.

Siintola, E., Lehesjoki, A. -E. and Mole, S. E. (2006) Molecular genetics of the NCLs–Status and perspectives. *Biochimicaet Biophysica Acta*. 1762: 857–64.

Thompson, J. B. (1991) Editor's Introduction. In: *Language and Symbollic Power*, P. Bourdieu, Cambridge: Polity.

Wainwright, D. (1996) The Political Transformation of the Health Inequalities Debate. *Critical Social Policy*. 16: 67–82.

Williams, S. J. (1995) Theorising, Class, Health and Lifestyles: Can Bourdieu help us? *Sociology of Health and Illness*. 52 (5): 577–604.

6 Merleau-Ponty, medicine and the body

Nick Crossley

Of all areas of sociological enquiry medicine most clearly involves 'the body'. Medical practices address the body in sickness and, increasingly, also in health, and they are themselves embodied: through the sensory experience and physical interventions of medical professionals. Medical knowledge is knowledge of bodies gleaned by way of embodied intervention; that is, intervention by a 'body' on a body. And medical practice is embodied practice; again practice upon bodies by bodies, involving an ensemble of (body) techniques of looking, listening, touching, manipulating, etc.

The importance of the work of Merleau-Ponty for medical sociology stems from this fact. He is, above all, a philosopher of embodiment. Specifically, his work is important for medical sociology in four key respects.

First, he offers a detailed philosophical account of 'the body' that, I will suggest, challenges the biologically reductive accounts sometimes found in medicine and allied disciplines, but without falling into the problems of idealism and relativism sometimes incurred by constructionist approaches in the social sciences.

Second, although he insists that we are our bodies and that our embodiment is the key to our experience, he argues that our embodiment is in some ways a blind spot for us, escaping our perception and reflection – a thesis further developed by Leder (1990). I will suggest that this observation sheds light upon bodily and specifically health-related activities and omissions that are otherwise difficult to account for from a sociological perspective, especially given the heightened body and health consciousness that we are supposed to be experiencing in late modernity (Giddens 1990).

Third, the absence of the body from everyday experience also provides an important backdrop for understanding illness experience. As Leder, building upon Merleau-Ponty, notes, illness lifts the body from the background of our experience to the foreground; the body *dys-appears*, with significant consequences in terms of both our personal identity and our capacity to engage with the world.

Finally, Merleau-Ponty offers an account of embodied practice that could form a useful basis from which to reflect upon and analyse medical practices. Even in the world of hi-tech medicine, medical intervention is a craft and involves embodied work. As such it can be illuminated by Merleau-Ponty's reflections upon embodied knowledge and understanding.

In what follows I discuss each of these points in turn. I begin with Merleau-Ponty's conception of the body.

Flesh and blood

In the conclusion to his seminal work on the sociology of the body, *Body and Society*, Brian Turner (1984) concedes that he feels less clear about the nature of the body at the end of his reflections than when he first began. What, he invites us to ask, is 'the body'? Such comments and questions can sound absurd. Bodies are hard, physical objects that we encounter and bump into, metaphorically if not literally, with startling frequency on a daily basis. They have parts (heart, lungs, liver, skin, bones) that are all connected and whose combination constitutes a living system; a system that sometimes goes wrong and requires medical intervention. Surely we know what the body is?

Turner is not persuaded, however, and he is not alone. Social constructionists, beginning with Foucault (1973), have questioned the adequacy of both this commonsense, 'flesh and blood' account and the more sophisticated formulation that it receives within medical discourse. The body is a 'construction', they argue, with apparent critical intent. Different cultures and eras perceive and conceive of bodies very differently. Such critiques are often far from convincing. It is true that representations of the body change over time and vary between cultures but that does not alter the fact that some representations are better than others, at least for specified purposes; an observation that tends to undermine the critical intent of the constructionist. And the critique is further undermined by the fact that constructionist epistemology deems all representations constructions, such that claims to this effect in any given case are of little consequence. Furthermore, whatever their arguments regarding variable conceptions, the constructionist struggles to explain away the perceptible self-evidence of bodies, illness and pain; that is, they struggle with flesh and blood. Indeed, the very fact of different conceptions of the body tends to suggest a shared underlying object of experience that different cultures, nevertheless, construct differently. For all of this, however, the biomedical construction of the body and its everyday 'flesh and blood' counterpart are not beyond critique.

Merleau-Ponty encounters the 'flesh and blood' conception of the body in the work of Descartes, where it is coupled with an immaterial mind in a bigger, if ultimately incoherent conception of the human being. Mind and body are two distinct 'substances' for Descartes. And the substance of the body or 'matter', since he is not only interested in human bodies but in all physical being ('bodies' in the Newtonian sense), is characterised by five key properties:

1 It extends into space.
2 It can be divided into ever smaller parts: e.g. in mortuary dissection, a practice in which Descartes participated and which fascinated him (Leder 1998).
3 It (only) moves in virtue of the application of external force to it.

4 It obeys deterministic laws (e.g. of motion) that can be uncovered by science. It is not without relevance in this respect that Descartes' key work, the *Meditations*, was published in 1641, one year before Galileo died and Newton was born. Neither is it without relevance that he had a fascination for clockwork toys, which move like human bodies when human beings transfer energy to them by winding them up (ibid.).
5. It is known by way of external perception. We know bodies because and to the extent that we can see them, touch them, prod them, hear, smell and even taste them. Descartes' own abovementioned education in the mortuary is relevant again here. He and his contemporaries were learning a great many new things about the human body by looking, touching, prodding, cutting, etc., a point whose later significance for medical knowledge is noted by Foucault (1973) amongst others. Western science only came to know life, in the form of the body, Foucault argues, by means of death; by 'open[ing] up a few corpses', to take a chapter title from *Birth of the Clinic*.

The properties of 'mind' qua substance are more or less the inverse of those of the body for Descartes.

1 Minds do not extend into space.
2 They are indivisible.
3 Their action is not a mere effect of external forces upon them.
4 They do not obey the laws of the physical universe.
5 They cannot be known by means of external perception (as non-spatial substances they have no outside). Rather they are known immediately, from within, by means of introspection.
6 More positively, minds think and this defines them qua substance. The mind is a thinking substance.

Minds are primary for Descartes. My mind is the essence of who I am. My body is to some degree accidental and inessential. He claims, for example, to be able to imagine that his body is an illusion and does not really exist without thereby imagining that he himself does not exist. Descartes cannot imagine his own non-existence because the very act of imagining presupposes that existence, but he can, he claims, imagine himself without a body. Indeed, it is his ability to 'doubt' the existence of his body (for philosophical and methodological purposes) without thereby doubting his own existence per se that first convinces him of the real and substantial distinction between mind and body. If Descartes can imagine himself existing without his body then his essence must lie elsewhere than his body.

Cartesian dualism has been criticised many times over from many different perspectives (see Carruthers 1986 for an overview). Usually such critiques focus upon 'the mind', arguing in different ways that it is not a separate substance from the body. Merleau-Ponty (1962), however, like Husserl (1970, 1973, 1989) before him, focuses at least as much upon 'the body'. Descartes' body, both argue, is an abstraction. This sounds counterintuitive. What could be more concrete than the body that Descartes describes; a body that we can see, touch, prod, cut open, etc.? What Merleau-Ponty and Husserl mean, however, is that Descartes' definition and understanding of the body focuses only upon certain of its properties. Indeed, it abstracts just those properties that can be seen, touched, prodded and opened up. As such it frames the body as an external object. The body, for Descartes, is something that stands (or lies) before him, passively, an object of knowledge or potential object of knowledge that he, qua subject, can come to know as such.

What is missing here is any consideration of the embodiment of the act and experience of perception itself. Seeing, touching and smelling the body of the other or any other object is itself an embodied experience. It requires that 'my body' makes contact with or at least comes into range of their body, but no less importantly my very perceptual consciousness is sensuous and embodied. We experience the world, perceptually, by means of (physical) sensations. The truth of this can sometimes be overlooked on account of the *intentionality* of perceptual experiences (Leder 1990). Perception is always of something and it is the something that we are aware of, not the perceptual sensations themselves. To see the computer before me I must have visual sensations but I do not perceive the sensations. They constitute a background against which the computer itself stands in the foreground as the object of my perception. The embodied basis of the perceptual experience can be brought home to us, however, when the objects we perceive overwhelm us in some way: e.g. when bright lights hurt our eyes, loud noise hurts our ears or a foul smell makes us feel sick (ibid.). In these cases the gestalt shifts, bringing the background to the foreground and vice versa; we lose our perceptual grip or focus upon the external object and lose any sense of its meaning because our experience has become focused upon the sensations (the pain or sickness) themselves.

Perceptual experiences reveal what both Husserl (1973, 1989) and Merleau-Ponty (1962) refer to as 'the other side' of the body. The body is a potential object of perception, it can be seen, heard, touched, smelled and tasted, but it is also and equally a sensuous being that experiences the world around it by means of sight, sound, touch, taste and smell. These are not 'add ons' to the body or secondary in any way. They are as much a part of what bodies are as the 'objective' properties identified by Descartes, and his conception of the body is not in any way more fundamental. It is one-sided and incomplete; an abstraction. It has proved to be a useful abstraction in many respects but it is no less an abstraction for that.

And however useful it may have been it has also been damaging in the respect that, over time and for many of us, its status as an abstraction has been overlooked. It has come to be seen as an exhaustive account of what the body is or at least an account of what is most fundamental about the body. The body has been reduced to its sense perceptible aspect; to an external object of perception. Its subjective, sensuous aspect has been displaced.

This, in some part, explains Descartes' dualism and the philosophical problems it creates. It is because he defines the body as he does, namely, as a sense perceptible object and nothing more, that Descartes is forced to invoke a further 'substance', mind, to incorporate subjective experience and the knowing subject in his account. It is often argued that Descartes' dualism reflects his divided loyalty to religion, on one side, and the newly emerging (materialist) science of his day, on the other. This is no doubt true. But even without a conception of the soul to somehow reconcile with his rather crude conception of bodies, the very crudeness of that conception clearly fails to encompass all that was given to Descartes' experience, and calls for him to map out another realm in which the excluded aspects of his experience, and indeed the fact of his experiencing anything at all, can be located. It is little wonder that Descartes identifies his essence outside of his body given his abstract and reductive account of the body.

This critique resonates with that of Gilbert Ryle (1949), who claims that Cartesian dualism is founded upon a category error. That we have different concepts for and discourses of 'mental' and 'physical' phenomena does not mean that they refer to distinct things, Ryle argues, any more than 'Queen', 'wife of Prince Philip' and 'head of the Church of England' refer to different people. Rather, they abstract different qualities from the same thing. Descartes' mistake is failing to recognise this. The different vocabularies of mind and matter confuse him into believing that mind and body are distinct substances.

The phenomenology of embodiment

The phenomenology of embodiment, beginning with Husserl (1973, 1989) but finding full expression in Merleau-Ponty (1962), challenges Descartes' reductive account and replaces it with a richer account rooted in a rigorous reflection upon human experience. Descartes follows the path that he does, Husserl notes, because he takes the scientific definition of matter, as formulated by Galileo, for granted in his account. Descartes claims to discover the separation of body from mind when discovering that he can doubt the existence of his body without thereby doubting his own existence but, Husserl argues, he can only doubt the existence of his body, without thereby doubting his own existence, because he is already thinking about his body in reductive terms, as mere matter; an external object of perception. This becomes obvious when he describes the properties of the body. Ignoring the sensuousness that a genuinely radical and unprejudiced reflection would have identified, he uncritically regurgitates Galileo's definition of matter. His reflection fails to reach behind the constructs of the educated public of his day and merely reiterates them.

The problem here is methodological. Descartes intended his *Meditations* as a radical philosophical reflection. He wanted to establish a solid foundation for the emerging science of his day. To that end he elected to suspend his habitual adherence to its claims and indeed to doubt anything of which he could not be absolutely certain. He would conduct a radical interrogation of his own experience in search of an 'Archimedean point' of certainty upon which to found knowledge. In taking Galileo's definition of matter for granted he fails in this task. He draws upon scientific ideas in his very attempt to ground science, rendering his position circular. More importantly (for our purposes), he fails to conduct a proper, radical philosophical interrogation of 'the body'.

Husserl's (later) phenomenology and a fortiori Merleau-Ponty's are intended as a corrective to this. Phenomenology is the radical reflection upon experience that

Descartes aimed for but failed to achieve. This reflection famously brackets out claims regarding the 'real' existence of objects beyond experience – not because phenomenologists doubt that existence in the sense Descartes' claims to do[1] – but more importantly it also seeks to get beneath the many conceptual abstractions through which we routinely 'construct' the world to explore the world as lived: the lived world or lifeworld.[2]

The body is integral to this. The phenomenologists seek to get beneath Descartes' abstract concept of matter in a full exploration of the 'lived body'. Husserl (1973, 1989) sets the ball rolling, claiming that a radical and unprejudiced interrogation of his experience reveals the embodiment of that experience and the 'other side' of the body noted above. His primordial consciousness of the world, perceptual consciousness, comprises a structure of lived bodily feelings. Merleau-Ponty (1962) further develops and elaborates on this at length, exploring these perceptual processes by way of an interrogation of lived experience. Moreover, he extends the challenge to Descartes' 'external' perspective upon the body by showing, contra Descartes, that his experiences of both his own body and the bodies of others are quite unlike that of his experience of external objects. This point needs to be unpacked.

Dealing first with perception, Merleau-Ponty, following Sartre's (1969) lead, notes that his body is his vantage point upon the world. Perception is always perception from somewhere (e.g. above, the side, a distance, close up), and necessarily so. There could be no perception without perspective. Our body is quite different to any other vantage point from which we might experience the world, however, such as a cliff top that affords us a vantage point upon the sea. We can always step back from the cliff top, ceasing to use it as a vantage point and making it an object of our perception, an object upon which we have a vantage point. We can never step back from our body, however. We can never escape the perspective it affords. It is the vantage point upon which there can be no vantage point; the vanishing point to which our perception is indissociably wedded. In this respect our body is quite unlike the external perceptible objects of our experience. A radical reflection upon our experience reveals that our body is not an object of perception but rather a condition of the possibility of our perceiving anything. Consciousness is, in the first instance, perceptual consciousness and perceptual consciousness is an articulation of body and world.

Similarly, again following Sartre (1969) and resonating with Mauss (1979), Merleau-Ponty notes that our bodies can be thought of as tools or instruments, but only if we recognise an important respect in which they are fundamentally different from all other tools. In order to use most tools I must do something and we can describe what it is that I do. In order to use a saw, for example, I must pick it up by the handle, grip it firmly in my hand, hold the wood that I am to saw with my other hand, etc. Likewise, to drive the car I must grasp the key in my hand, put the key in the ignition, turn it, press the clutch pedal, etc. I can give no comparable account in relation to my body however. I do not do anything to my body in order to move it. It just moves, or rather I move. I am tempted to say that it moves in the way that I intend but this must not be interpreted to mean that my body obeys an intention or follows an order that somehow precedes it. In the normal everyday case, moving and intending to move are the same. 'Intention' is a property of my movement, not an independent or antecedent cause of it. My movements are not planned, prepared or thought about. I do not know how I do them, and again that is perhaps because 'I' do not exist apart from them. I am them. I am a body and my body is an active, moving being; always already in motion and in constant interaction with its perceived surround.

The body of the other seems, prima facie, to correspond more closely to the external object that Descartes describes, but here too Merleau-Ponty disagrees. Perception, in its most primordial form, he maintains, is not objectification but rather communication: a search for meaning and an interaction (on various levels). The other is not a body but rather embodies meanings in her actions and gestures that move me to respond in like fashion. I no more experience a body when face to face with the other than I experience physical markings on paper when reading a book. As with the book my perception takes me beyond sheer physical being to its meaning, a meaning that I may step back from to contemplate but that, in the first instance, absorbs and mobilises me into a response. I am moved by the other; moved into action and gesture by the meanings that her actions and gestures communicate to me. And much of this happens without reflective awareness or intervention: a smile elicits a smile. I respond to the other before and without aid of any reflection that may subsequently take place. To objectify the other is to refuse this communication and step back from it.

Feminist critics, such as Young (1980), have responded to such claims by arguing that Merleau-Ponty fails to account for the objectification of the female body. Moreover, they suggest that such objectification, particularly when internalised by women, effects a very different experience of embodiment to that described by Merleau-Ponty, such that his is effectively an account of masculine embodiment and not the universal account he purports to offer. Young notes that women's awareness of the objectification of their bodies by men alienates them from their bodies and inhibits their capacity for smooth and spontaneous action. Action is smooth and spontaneous when habitual, in Merleau-Ponty's sense (see below), but much less so when actors, made aware of themselves through their awareness of the voyeurism of others and the need to defend themselves against unwanted attention, must think about how they act. Objectification of women's bodies prevents women from feeling fully 'at home' in their bodies and inhibits their capacity for spontaneous and pre-reflective action. Furthermore, women learn ways of acting that anticipate and pre-empt unwanted attention, which are often also more awkward than their male equivalents (but see Young 1998, Grimshaw 1999).

This criticism is important but so too is Merleau-Ponty's underlying point, and it retains a universal element even if gendered and other variations are not properly thought through in relation to it. Others communicate to us by means of their actions and gestures, even when not meaning to, and this is what is most often striking, what is at the foreground, in our encounters with them. The flesh and bones of the Cartesian body only come to the foreground when these meanings are prevented from surfacing. Perhaps it should not surprise us that Descartes learned of bodies through the mortuary. His body is a dead body.

The medical body

How does any of this relate to medical sociology and to my introductory remarks on social construction, aside perhaps from the fact that medics too, at least traditionally, learn their trade with dead bodies? Merleau-Ponty's reflections, in my view, lend philosophical depth to the claims of the constructionists. The biological models of the body adhered to in much medicine, which represent the contemporary form of the Cartesian conception, are not wrong but they are abstractions that, qua abstractions, are partial and which simplify. They draw certain aspects of the body to the foreground of our attention and knowledge, pushing others into the background. For this reason they are not fundamental. They do not represent the bottom line. They capture only one aspect of something much more complex and multi-faceted. This sense of construction as abstraction lends some critical weight to the notion of 'construction' without requiring that constructions need all be equivalent, or having to deny that they 'work'. Biological constructions of the body may prove more or less useful in guiding our attempts to alleviate pain, disease, etc., but we should never forget that they are abstractions and that, as such, they foreground certain aspects of the body at the expense of others that are, in other ways, equally important.

This contention also supports those who seek a more holistic approach in medicine but not those who do so by means of simple addition: e.g. those who argue for a bio + psycho + social model. Descartes recognised that 'the body' alone does not suffice to account for human being and sought to add 'mind' to it. He might equally have added 'society' too. But this additive approach can remain locked in the category error described by Ryle (1949), treating different aspects of human existence as if they were different things or parts; an endeavour that always ends in sticky disputes as to how such different parts can belong to the same whole in any integrated fashion. Merleau-Ponty, by contrast, offers a philosophically robust argument that the 'parts' are not parts at all but rather aspects, abstractions from an underlying, undifferentiated whole. Biology, psychology and social life are not separate things, not separate 'substances', but rather derive, qua objects of knowledge, from different ways of perceiving. And medical discourse is only able to construct its object by denying and repressing 'the other side' of the body.

This is not bad, in and of itself. It may be necessary. But the phenomenological critique unsettles the sense of naturalness, the taken for grantedness, that invests biological and 'flesh and blood' representations of the body. Furthermore, it highlights a moral aspect of inter-corporeal relations that is negated by the medical gaze. The objectification involved in medicine's construction of the body is not just the construction of a body but also a suspension of normal relations in which the bodies of ego and alter are entangled in communicative exchange. The medical gaze puts the 'expressive body' out of play in order to foreground 'the man machine', switching the gestalt and thereby suspending the normal moral order of inter-corporeal relations. The intersubjective relations that, for Merleau-Ponty, are primordial, are negated and replaced by a subject–object relation. Again this is not necessarily wrong. At the very least it most often has what all parties involved regard as a vital pragmatic utility. The patient will not be cured, at least from most illness, by talk. But it alerts us to a moral dimension of the medical encounter that might not otherwise come to light and warns us of a potential for danger, should this suspension of normal moral relations extend beyond what is useful.

Science and philosophy

Merleau-Ponty's critique of the scientific objectification of the body is extensive. For all of this, however, and in contrast to both Husserl and Heidegger, who recognise no place for the claims of science in their philosophy, Merleau-Ponty maintains a dialogue with science, particularly human science and more particularly still social science, in his work. His philosophy questions the assumptions, concepts and interpretations of science but at the same time insists that the philosopher can learn from science. Indeed, many of the central insights of his philosophy, particularly his early philosophy, are arrived at in a philosophical discussion and reworking of important experiments in psychology. The philosopher can sometimes see significance in scientific work that is not apparent to the scientist, he believes; but by the same token the empirical work of the scientist, whether medical or social scientific, can generate rigorous and counterintuitive observations that the philosopher would not arrive at by reflection and which cannot be ignored. Furthermore, he believes that social science, particularly in the form of gestalt psychology (which also informed the work of both E. Durkheim and G. H. Mead), converges with the key claims of phenomenological philosophy, generating an opportunity for genuine dialogue.

This is nowhere more apparent than in *The Structure of Behaviour*, a work that pre-dates his full-blown engagement with phenomenology but informs it, and which explores scientific knowledge of the body, in the form of 'the organism', in some depth. Two key claims from this work are worthy of brief mention.

First, Merleau-Ponty mounts a powerful critique of the 'clockwork' view of bodily activity that runs back from (Pavlovian) behaviourism to Descartes. The experiments of the behaviourists fail to bear out their theory, he observes, suggesting rather that human and other higher organisms are animated by purposes and interact with their environment on the basis of the meaning it assumes for them. 'Stimuli' do not 'cause' action via 'reflex arcs'. Rather, objects and events are responded to on the basis of their significance and how they fit with the goals of the organism.

Second, he argues for a holistic view of human and animal life in which consciousness and other 'mental' phenomena are interpreted not, à la Descartes, as facets of a separate substance but rather as emergent phenomena arising from interactions both within the organism and between organism and environment. Consciousness is not a 'thing' from this point of view but rather a 'relation' arising from interaction between organism and environment and residing between them. Similarly, the language of cognition, emotion, etc., refers not to ghostly goings on in an immaterial realm but rather to forms of embodied conduct and experience directed at and deriving their meaning and identity from specific environmental contexts.

Interestingly, from our point of view, the need for a holistic interpretation is no more apparent for Merleau-Ponty than in cases where the body suffers some form of lesion. The effect, he argues, is often only poorly captured by an atomistic account in which localised lesions have localised effects. Rather, the organism typically adjusts to and compensates for the lesion, resulting in effects across the system and not just within a single organ or bodily part.

These arguments, first introduced in *The Structure of Behaviour*, are returned to repeatedly in Merleau-Ponty's major work, *The Phenomenology of Perception*, as is one poor unfortunate, Schneider, whose well-documented symptoms following a head injury serve to illustrate much that Merleau-Ponty wants to argue. Schneider's abnormal experience provides an entry point for Merleau-Ponty's phenomenological exploration of normal experience. It affords him a fascinating point of contrast from which to explore human consciousness and experience. Merleau-Ponty is always mindful to remind his reader, however, that Schneider's difficulties are not symbolic in origin but organic. He received an injury to his brain. 'Medical' problems may derive from purposive, embodied agency for Merleau-Ponty, as psychosomatic and hysterical symptoms suggest, but nothing that we say about the 'subjective side' of the body negates the fact of its 'objective side'. The phenomenology of the body-subject is no more exhaustive of 'the body' than the science of the body-object; these two perspectives are sides of a coin. Moreover, illness and injury may be just the experiences that require us to switch the gestalt and explore the body's object-side. I return to this point later.

Reflexivity and the bodily blind spot

We are our bodies, for Merleau-Ponty. My body is my way of being-in-the-world. My bodily action does not reflect my volition. Under normal circumstances it is my volition. And qua consciousness I am embodied consciousness, a sensuous grasp upon the world. Perhaps counter-intuitively, however, this very fact tends to make my body, to borrow Leder's term, 'absent' from my own experience:

> For myself I am neither 'jealous', nor 'inquisitive', nor 'hunchbacked', nor 'a civil servant'. It is often a matter of surprise that the cripple can put up with himself. The reason is that for themselves such people are neither deformed nor at death's door. Until the final coma the dying man is inhabited by a consciousness, he is all that he sees, and enjoys this much of an outlet. Consciousness can never objectify itself into invalid-consciousness or cripple-consciousness, and even if the old man complains of his age or the cripple of his deformity, they can only do so by comparing themselves with others, or seeing themselves through the eyes of others, that is by taking a statistical or objective view of themselves …
>
> (Merleau-Ponty 1962: 434)

The above passage suggests two reasons for this absence. The first is that experience, to reiterate an earlier point, is 'intentional'; consciousness is always necessarily consciousness of something outside of itself. My perception of the computer before me consists of a pattern of sensations but I am not conscious of the sensations. I am conscious of the computer. I am, to paraphrase Merleau-Ponty, all that I see. Embodied consciousness projects me outside of myself, into the world. It gives me a world. If the sensation were to be foregrounded in my experience then the world would recede into the background. I would cease to be aware of it. Similarly, in acting I do not focus upon my actions but rather on the world in which I am acting. When driving, for example, I do not attend to what my feet and hands are doing but rather to the road. And good thing too! Not only do I need to attend to the road if I am to avoid crashing, but attending to my actions would inhibit them, rendering them awkward and clumsy – much as Young says of women's bodily experience (see above). My body is absent from my experience, in this sense, because I am focused outside of myself, upon the world.

Second, I only have my own experience and, in the first instance at least, therefore have no comparison against which to judge it different, deficient or indeed to get any kind of perspective upon it. If male experience is in some way different to female experience, to take one example, I have no way of knowing that from my experience itself because all I know is the world as I experience it.

This applies equally, to some extent, to my perception of my bodily exterior. Being tall does not make me feel tall and I can only feel tall or short or fat or thin by comparing myself with others who differ from me. Indeed, this is not only a matter of how I feel. Within certain bounds there is no standard of human 'tallness' other than that provided by the statistical norm (and that norm will vary historically in accordance with diet).

Merleau-Ponty insists that I can only experience my body, as such, if I can achieve an external perspective upon it and I can only do this by learning to perceive myself from the 'perspective of other', to borrow Mead's (1967) phrase. Only by imagining ourselves from the outside, as others see us, can we truly exist for ourselves as objects of experience. Reflexivity is therefore an emergent property of social interaction and relations.

When we have achieved this capacity for reflection, however, changes across time too may afford us the comparative framework necessary to put our experiences into perspective. My deteriorating eyesight and need for glasses was revealed to me when I found myself struggling to read small print that I once read with ease, for example. There was nothing in my eyesight itself that indicated deterioration. I began to wear glasses much later than I should have because I didn't realise that I had become short sighted. But a comparison of my former and present abilities, coupled with a sense that others saw better than me, did eventually bring the problem to light.

As this example also suggests, however, where change is slow a habitual shift in expectations may obscure this opportunity for insight. If my eyesight fades over time then I am less likely to notice deterioration. My expectations about what I am capable of shift with my eyesight. Without really noticing it, for example, I acquire the habit of standing closer to signs in order to read them.

This applies equally to changes in our external appearance. The mirror affords me regular and frequent access to my external appearance; too regular and frequent to allow me to notice gradual changes. My perceptual expectations about myself shift slowly, on a daily basis, along with my appearance. As long as nothing happens too suddenly I am not forced to notice. Likewise with close friends, whose bodily changes escape our notice because our perceptual expectations of them change with them. It is for this reason that we are often shocked to see the change in old friends we have not seen for a while, but much less aware of the changes in those with whom we spend regular time.

These blind spots go some way to explaining why early signs of serious illness and more especially the effects of unhealthy lifestyles pass unnoticed for extended periods, and why such lifestyle patterns tend to cluster. The actor accommodates to gradual changes. Nothing in their experience gives them the vantage point from which to recognise the changes they are undergoing.

Weight gain is an obvious example. Actors often express shock at having discovered the excess weight they have put on over time. There may be a rhetorical element to this – shock sounds better than admitting to a previous lack of concern – but Merleau-Ponty's perspective, as outlined above, suggests that gradual bodily change may well pass unnoticed, especially if those in the actor's reference group have adjusted over time to the changes and are changing in similar ways themselves.

It may seem odd to be discussing the absence of the body from experience in an era of such heightened body consciousness as our own. Sociology teaches us that the combined effect of consumption and the rise of the 'bio-political' state has been to heighten bodily consciousness as never before (Crossley 2006). The dramatic rise of obesity and of people being overweight suggests that we are not as vigilant about our bodies as some sociological accounts suggest, however. And Merleau-Ponty's account is important because it points to the difficulties that we may have in achieving an objective vantage point upon our body in the absence of objectifying interventions (e.g. regularly weighing ourselves and taking our measurements). Our bodies are always in some respect a blind spot for us according to Merleau-Ponty.

Illness and bodily dys-appearance

At least they are until we become ill. As Leder (1990) notes acute illness and pain bring the body into sharp relief. The body becomes thematic in experience when it ceases to work as normal or when its sensations are intense and painful. Dysfunction makes the body appear to itself. The body *dys-appears*.

This makes the experience of illness unsettling. It brings that which ordinarily belongs to the background of experience to the foreground, reminding actors of the embodied basis of their being-in-the-world and perhaps also thereby their mortality. All that they ordinarily take for granted is revealed to them as dependent upon their body, which at the very moment of realising this they also experience as vulnerable. And there are two further aspects to this unsettling experience. First, shifting the focus of experience onto the body tends to focus it away from the world. Illness is therefore, in some part, a retreat from the world in a very fundamental sense. The embodied agent is less able to project themselves into the world, as they ordinarily do. Their experience is thrown back upon itself. Likewise pain can shrink the actor's lived world, again focusing them in upon their self and inhibiting their focus on the world beyond.

Second, this disruption of what is ordinarily taken for granted involves a disruption of the actor's habitual sense of both their body and world (see also below). Although not ordinarily reflectively conscious of their body in everyday activity, the actor nevertheless has a habitual sense of what they are capable of doing, which they draw upon in confronting situations, and indeed a habitual understanding and knowledge of the world, born of experience (see below). Illness, by undermining the powers of the body, undermines this habitual sense and the confidence (or ontological security) that attaches to it. The actor may lose confidence in or become unsure of their bodily abilities, again forcing the body to the foreground of experience and again, therefore, shrinking their world.

Illness experiences are an important focus of medical sociology, and Merleau-Ponty and Leder provide a useful resource for thinking further upon them. Importantly, however, we must be careful not to slip into the assumption that the actor's illness experiences are unmediated. Our experience of ourselves, as noted earlier, is always mediated through others and as such it reflects the wider culture to which we belong. The embodied subject is never transparent to herself and in seeking to make sense of experiences that she finds disturbing she will draw upon dominant cultural constructions:

> The adult himself will discover in his own life what his culture, education, books and tradition have taught him to find there. The contact I make with myself is always mediated by a particular culture, or at least by a language that we have received from without and which guides us in our self-knowledge.
> (Merleau-Ponty 2004: 86–87)

This point is made against Descartes' claim that 'the mind' is transparent to itself; that it knows itself 'immediately'. It applies equally to embodied experience, however, and a fortiori to the body 'beneath the skin'. Each actor has their own unique bodily experience, but in the effort to make sense of such experiences they must draw upon a shared stock of culture, including, of course, medical knowledge. The actor experiences her body through the frame provided by medical discourse.

This brings us back, on one level, to a form of constructionism. It suggests the need for a critical engagement with constructionism, however, insofar as it identifies an underlying experience of pain or disease that calls for such interpretation. One is reminded on this point of Canguilhem's (1998) contention that we do not feel ill because we have medical categories and knowledge but rather have medical categories and knowledge because we sometimes feel ill. The first condition of the body having become an object of knowledge, Canguilhem insists, is what he calls the breaking of the 'silence of the organs'. That is to say, the body has become an object of medical knowledge, in the first instance, because the experience of illness has drawn it across an epistemological threshold.

Leder's arguments about bodily dys-appearance, and the ideas of Merleau-Ponty which they draw upon, illuminate this process at the phenomenological level. They show how, in illness, the body becomes thematic to itself and thereby available for objectification and observation. Illness, as I noted earlier, effects a gestalt switch, bringing the body to the foreground of experience. Canguilhem (1998), and his student, Foucault (1973), pick up the story from this point, considering just how the body is objectified and constructed in medical practice. It is only against the background of the earlier phenomenological account, to pick up a central thread of this chapter, however, that their research has any critical import.

Embodied medical practice

All that I have said so far has focused upon 'the body' on the receiving end of medicine. Medicine is itself embodied, however. It is a social practice, comprising bodily activities and techniques. Merleau-Ponty has nothing to say about these practices, as such, but he has much to offer our attempts to understand embodied practice more generally. In what remains of this chapter I will outline one key contribution to the understanding of practice that his work affords; his concept of habit.

Habit, for Merleau-Ponty, is practical knowledge and understanding – what Ryle (1949) calls 'know-how'. To acquire a habit is to acquire a new way of handling the world, a new way of perceiving and mastering some aspect of it that, necessarily, bestows fresh (practical) meaning upon it. And it is necessarily embodied: 'We say that the body has understood and habit been cultivated when it has absorbed a new meaning and assimilated a fresh core of significance' (Merleau-Ponty 1962: 146).

We said earlier that it is the body that understands in the acquisition of habit. This way of putting it will appear absurd, if understanding is subsuming a sense datum under an idea, and if the body is an object. But the phenomenon of habit is just what prompts us to revise our notion of 'understand' and our notion of the body. To understand is to experience harmony between what we aim at and what is given, between intention and the performance – and the body is our anchorage in the world (ibid.: 144).

If habit is neither a form of knowledge nor an involuntary action what then is it? It is knowledge in the hands that is forthcoming only when bodily effort is made, and cannot be formulated in detachment from that effort. The subject knows where the letter, are on the typewriter as we know where one of our limbs is, through knowledge bred of familiarity that does not give us a position in objective space (ibid.).

My hands deploy a practical knowledge of key positions when I type, for example, and they subordinate the space of the keyboard to my purpose, bestowing a meaning upon it. Likewise the doctor conducting an examination, performing surgery or operating a machine. The tools of medicine are tools only for hands trained to use them as such. In untrained hands they have no use and therefore no meaning, or at least they do not have the same use as they have for the doctor and therefore cannot have the same meaning.

This is a matter of motor activity but equally also of perception. Medical hands, ears and eyes are trained to interrogate bodies, talk and machine outputs in search of what, to their tutored receptivity, are signs of illness and health:

> In the gaze we have at our disposal a natural instrument akin to the blind man's stick. The gaze gets more or less out of things according to the way in which it questions them, ranges over or dwells on them. To learn to see colours is to acquire a new style of seeing, a new use of one's own body; it is to enrich and recast the body image.
>
> (Merleau-Ponty 1962: 157)

The embodiment of medical practice is nowhere more evident than in the acquired perceptual schemas of practitioners, and the medical gaze, in its most literal form, is embodied in the perceptual experience of the medical practitioner.

Picking up another of Merleau-Ponty's arguments, moreover, the tools of the doctor's trade become an extension of her body. Like the blind man's stick referred to in the above passage, for example, the stethoscope is not a perceptual object for the doctor but rather an extension of her body and, specifically, of her perceptual capacities. She does not hear it but rather hears with it. Similarly, the tools of surgery become an extension of the surgeon's hands and are incorporated within her tacit, embodied sense of herself. Just as the accomplished driver takes the size and speed of the car into account, tacitly, when parking or pulling into traffic, so too the accomplished keyhole surgeon incorporates the dimensions of their instruments when operating, becoming one with the tool in order to use it effectively.

These observations are speculative and only scratch at the surface, but hopefully they say enough to indicate that Merleau-Ponty's investigation of embodiment has something to offer an investigation of the embodiment of medical practice. And this is important. The source of Descartes' error in relation to the body was focusing only upon the body of the other, the external body, at the expense of a proper reflection upon his own embodiment and the embodied conditions that gave rise to his perception of other bodies. We should not make the same mistake with respect to medicine. The body is both the subject and the object in medical practice.

Conclusion

One cannot venture far in medical sociology without coming into contact with bodies. On first glance these bodies might seem fairly straightforward and obvious entities, rather more concrete than much we encounter in sociology. They are not, however, and the value of Merleau-Ponty's perspective is that it allows us to explore and reflect upon the body in ways that are at once philosophically challenging and useful. Specifically, Merleau-Ponty alerts us to the 'lived body', excluded equally in Cartesian, medical and constructionist accounts. He reminds us that we are our bodies whilst simultaneously explaining why that tends to make our bodies a blind spot, a fact that helps to explain both why we are ignorant of so much about our bodies and also why illness can have such a profound effect upon our sense of ourselves. Finally, and no less importantly, he provides us with some basic tools by which to begin thinking of the embodiment of medical practice itself.

Notes

1 Husserl and Merleau-Ponty differ on this point. Husserl (1990) maintains that it is impossible to prove the existence of the world beyond consciousness because any such proof would necessarily rely upon the evidence of consciousness and would therefore be circular. He also maintains, however, that it makes no sense to doubt that which cannot be proven either way. The world beyond consciousness is not in any doubt in Husserl's philosophy therefore. Merleau-Ponty (1962) accepts this but also points to the various ways in which 'the real' seemingly thwarts our attempts to impose meaning and order upon it. What we learn from phenomenological reduction, he maintains, is its impossibility. In his philosophy, therefore, like that of Heidegger (1962) and Sartre (1969), the phenomenological bracketing of the 'external world' (reduction) is conceived as a way of better exploring our 'inherence in the world', a methodological conceit rather than a serious agnosticism.
2 The concept of the lifeworld is interpreted in different ways, partly because Husserl (1970) is uncharacteristically inconsistent in his use of it and also partly because of the different ways in which subsequent writers have developed it. This is one meaning of the concept, however.

References

Canguilhem, G. (1998) *The Normal and the Pathological*, New York, Zone.
Carruthers, P. (1986) *Introducing Persons*, London, Routledge.
Crossley, N. (2001a) *The Social Body: Habit, Identity and Desire*, London, Sage.
——(2001b) Merleau-Ponty, in Turner, B. and Elliott, A. (eds) *Profiles in Contemporary Social Theory*, London, Sage, 30–42
——(2006) *Reflexive Embodiment in Contemporary Society*, Buckinghamshire, Open University Press.
Foucault, M. (1973) *The Birth of the Clinic*, London, Tavistock.
Giddens, A. (1990) *Modernity and Self-Identity*, Cambridge, Polity.
Grimshaw, J. (1999) Working Out With Merleau-Ponty, in Arthurs, J. and Grimshaw, J. (eds) *Women's Bodies*, London, Cassell, 91–116.
Husserl, E. (1970) *The Crisis of the European Sciences and Transcendental Phenomenology*, Evanston, IL, Northwestern University Press.
——(1973) *Experience and Judgement*, Evanston, IL, Northwestern University Press.
——(1989) *Ideas Pertaining to a Pure Phenomenology and to a Phenomenological Philosophy (Second Book)*, Dordrecht, Kluwer.
—— (1990) *Cartesian Meditations*. Dordrecht, Kluwer.
Leder, D. (1990) *The Absent Body*, Chicago, Chicago University press.
——(1998) A Tale of Two Bodies, in Welton, D. (ed.) *Body and Flesh*, Oxford, Blackwell, 117–30.

Mauss, M. (1979) Body Techniques. In his *Sociology and Psychology*. London, Routledge.
Mead, G.-H. (1967) *Mind, Self and Society*, Chicago, Chicago University Press.
Merleau-Ponty, M. (1962) *The Phenomenology of Perception*, London, Routledge.
——(1965) *The Structure of Behaviour*, London, Methuen.
——(2004) *The World of Perception*, London, Routledge.
Ryle, G. (1949) *The Concept of Mind*, Harmondsworth, Penguin.
Turner, B. (1984) *Body and Society*, Oxford, Blackwell.
Young, I. (1980) Throwing Like a Girl, *Human Studies* 3, 137–56.
——(1998a) Throwing Like a Girl: Twenty Year On, in Weldon, D. (ed.) *Body and Flesh*, Oxford, Blackwell, 286–90.

7 World systems theory and the epidemiological transition

Martin Hyde and Anthony Rosie

Introduction

The American sociologist Immanuel Wallerstein (1930–) is a founding figure in world-system theory and research. Educated at Columbia University he completed a PhD on political systems in West Africa in the late 1950s. While he continued to write about Africa thereafter his attention moved to how Africa fitted into a larger world picture. The work of the historian Fernand Braudel (1993; 2002a; 2002b; 2002c), whose major study included an analysis of civilisation and capitalism, convinced Wallerstein of the need for both an analysis at the world-system level and a deep engagement with historical data. Rather than marking a radical change of direction, the emerging analysis of how lives are organised under a single world-system sought to contextualise all that Wallerstein had undertaken to the 1970s. His output since has been extensive and wide-ranging. However, his three volumes on the modern world-system are perhaps the most enduring part of his legacy. Published in 1974, 1980 and 1989, they chart the rise of a single, capitalist world-system from the late fifteenth century onwards. Through this work he argued that world-systems had replaced world-empires. However he was keen to stress that imperialism has not disappeared and that it remains relevant to the lives of many people around the globe.

Wallerstein's research into world-systems drew on Marx's analyses of production without being a Marxist theory. Braudel's civilisational analyses provided a mainspring and the Centre Wallerstein went on to found at Binghampton in 1979 was named in honour of Braudel. By the time he published the first volume of the history in 1974, Wallerstein was joining others in a critique of modernisation theory, the idea that if only 'less developed' countries did certain things borrowed from successful Western nations then they could have a brighter future. By 1974 the critiques of modernisation by dependency theorists such as Andre Gunder Frank and Fernando Cardoso, later the thirty-fourth president of Brazil, were becoming well known. Dependency theory posits that metropoles, or core areas, exert control through trade and other practices on peripheral nations through both the means of production and the cost of commodities.

One contribution Wallerstein made to this analysis was to point to the role of the semi-periphery, which acts to keep the other two components in place. The core areas act directly on both semi-periphery and periphery, but the expanding division of labour draws largely on the ways in which regions in the semi-periphery act directly on the periphery while also supporting the core. Of course if there is downward movement from countries in the core there is always a potential upward mover from the semi-periphery. The rise of China and India in the last 20 years provides an example.

Wallerstein remarked somewhat ruefully that students often read only the journal article he published in 1974 alongside the first volume of the history of the world-system. Certainly the journal article encapsulates the key arguments found across the three volumes, but a reader interested in how parts of the world were incorporated into the single world-system would need to read at least volume three of the history. Here the reader will find how West Africa was an external zone to the rising European capitalist system from the sixteenth to the eighteenth centuries, and how it was first peripheralised through the slave trade before becoming part of the periphery in the ever-strengthening single world-system.

Wallerstein's work provided a very real starting point for world-systems analysis. He sustained a wide range of inquiries from scholars all over the world, many coming to study at the Fernand Braudel Centre. Then the publication of journals and currently the *Journal of World-Systems Research* marked the establishment of the field as a point of reference in global sociology. As a convenor and then president of the International Sociological Association (ISA), Wallerstein has worked to bring together world social science scholarship in ways that are accessible to many.

World systems theory and epidemiological transition theory

Our aim in this chapter is to present an engagement between world systems theory (WST) and epidemiological transition theory (ETT). We believe that such an engagement has the potential to be mutually beneficial. Both are key theories in their field and have generated a vast amount of studies and reviews. However there has been no previous attempt to bring them together. This is surprising as both theories share a similar, macro-level, historical approach and take modernisation theory as their point of departure. Moreover each lacks what the other has to offer. Despite its interdisciplinary nature and the breadth of issues addressed by WST, there has been relatively little attention paid to population health, in particular fertility and mortality patterns, as a constituent part or expression of inequalities between states. Thus we hope to be able to draw world systems theorists' attention to the role that health might play, alongside economic and political factors, within a world system. ETT is also the focus of a host of varied and interdisciplinary studies. It has also become an increasingly key concept within the sociology of health and social epidemiology. However, like classic sociology in general, ETT suffers from a state-centric, methodologically nationalist, approach. Even when cross-national studies have been undertaken, nation-states are still represented as discreet units for comparison rather than being seen as interconnected parts of a whole. By definition a WST approach offers a crucial correction to this. This is the principle focus of our chapter. We wish to argue and to demonstrate that whilst the ETT offers an important framework to explore changes in the health of a population it is severely hampered by its neglect of the interconnections between states and the impact that they have on the epidemiological transition. Ultimately our central argument is relatively simple. It is that, contrary to the classic view of national trajectories through different epidemiological phases, population health is relational, insofar as the factors that determine it are part of a world system. We aim to show this through a mixture of macro-level data on trade and mortality patterns and a few brief comments on how the ideas might apply to the region of West Africa. However, before we can bring these two theories together it is necessary to describe their main components and criticisms for those who might be less familiar with either or both of them.

Epidemiological transition theory

Despite being largely overlooked when it was first proposed, Abdel Omran's (1971) epidemiological transition theory (ETT) has become something of a citation classic. The original paper has been cited nearly 600 times, although most of these are from the 1990s onwards and relatively few are found in epidemiology journals (Weisz and Olszynko-Gryn 2010). In this seminal paper Omran sought to set out

> [a] theory of epidemiologic transition [that is] sensitive to the formulations of population theorists who have stressed the demographic, biologic, sociologic, economic and psychologic (sic) ramifications of transitional processes ... Conceptually, the theory of epidemiologic transition focuses on the complex change in patterns of health and disease *and* on the interactions between these patterns and their demographic, economic and sociologic determinants and consequences.
>
> (Omran 1971: 510)

This theory has generated a great deal of research and support from around the world. Harper and Armelagos (2010: 667) applaud it for its

> focus on the population as the unit of study rather than the individual. This modification represents an important change in perspective that resulted from the influence of population biology on human disease ecology. Using the population as the unit of study allows us to move beyond the clinical perspective in order to consider diseases in their broader biological and social context.

It has also attracted criticism from a number of quarters. We will address these later along with our own. However one of the main weaknesses of the theory, its ambiguity, is also its strength. Omran's often frustrating lack of precision, about dates and the drivers of the transitions, and his rather eclectic use of theories and theorists means that the ETT is open to multiple readings. Weisz and Olszynko-Gryn (2010: 287) argue that it was 'part of a broader effort to reorient American and international health institutions towards the pervasive population control agenda of the 1960s and 1970s'. Others see it as an attempt to account for the 'extraordinary advances in health care made in industrialized countries since the 18th century' and focused on calculating maximum life expectancy (Caselli *et al.* 2002). Notwithstanding these interpretations Omran's work is now probably best known and employed as a way to explain the differences in the main causes of death, notably in the shift away from infectious diseases to chronic and degenerative diseases, between societies and over time. Mackenbach (1999: 329) observes that, despite its conceptual ambiguity,

> [t]he epidemiologic transition theory provides a potentially powerful framework for the study of disease and mortality in populations, especially for the study of historical and international variations.

It is this interpretation and the focus on the main causes of mortality that we will be using to assess the ETT in relation to the WST. Omran set out five propositions that underpin the ETT:

1 'The theory of epidemiologic transition begins with the major premise that mortality is a fundamental factor in population dynamics'(Omran 1971: 511).
2 'During the transition, a long term shift occurs in mortality and disease patterns whereby pandemics of infection are gradually displaced by degenerative and man-made diseases as the chief forms of morbidity and primary cause of death' (Omran 1971: 516).
3 'During the epidemiologic transition the most profound changes in health and disease patterns obtain among children and young women' (Omran 1971: 521).
4 'The shifts in health and disease patterns that characterize the epidemiologic transition are closely associated with the demographic and socioeconomic transition that constitute the modernization complex' (Omran 1971: 527).
5 'Peculiar variations in the pattern, the pace, the determinants and the consequences of population change differentiate three basic models of the epidemiologic transition: the classical or western model, the accelerated model and the contemporary or delayed model' (Omran 1971: 532).

In sum, he argues that as societies pass through successive stages of the modernisation process the main causes of mortality shift from infectious to chronic and degenerative diseases, which results in an increase in life expectancy and a decrease in fertility. The epidemiological transition in health and diseases is therefore closely associated with demographic and socioeconomic transition, and with changes in lifestyle and modernisation. As such, periods of human history ought to have a distinct mortality profile, and in turn one ought to be able to construct a periodisation of human history based on differing life expectancies and main causes of death.

He identifies three successive stages of the epidemiological transition. Table 7.1 outlines the main demographic, socio-economic and epidemiological characteristics

Table 7.1. The classic (Western) model

Transition Profiles	Age of Pestilence and Famine	Age of receding pandemics (early)
Population profile		
Population growth	The pattern of growth until about 1650 is cyclic with minimal increments: mortality dominates with crude death rates from 30 to more than 50/100 and with frequent higher peaks. Fertility is at a sustained high level of 40 or more per 1,000.	Mortality continues high (30–50 +/1,000) but peaks are less frequent and the general level begins declining. Fertility remains high (40+/1,000). The demographic gap widens somewhat, and there is a net population increase that, though small, is cumulative.
Population composition	The population is predominantly young, with large very young and small old dependency ratios and a slight excess of males. Residence is mainly rural with few crowded, unsanitary, war–famine–epidemic ridden cities of small or medium size.	The population is still young, though the proportion of older people begins to increase. The male–female ratio is near unity (100M/100F). Residence is still primarily rural but with a progressive exodus from farm to factory. Selective migration to new colonies relieves population pressure somewhat in home countries but upsets the age–sex composition.
Economic profile	Subsistence economies characterise agrarian societies, which depend on manual, labour-intensive production methods. Occasional breakthroughs and sporadic rises in wages are largely undermined by low incentives and cosmic catastrophes while labour efficiency is marred by debilitative diseases.	Preconditions for economic 'take-off' appear: improvements in agriculture and land-use coupled with modest development of transportation–communication networks encourage industrialisation; leading sectors of production, e.g. textiles and lumber, emerge.
Social profile		
Society	Society is traditional with a fatalistic orientation sustained by rigid, hierarchical socio-political structures.	A traditional/provincial outlook persists among the lower classes while the upper and emerging middle classes of businessmen adopt 'faith in reason'.
Family and women	Clan or extended family structures with large family size, multiple generation households and home centred lifestyles are dominant. Women are cast strictly in the mother role with virtually no rights or responsibilities outside the home.	Extended family systems and large family size still prevail. The maternal role begins to allow a little involvement in such areas as home crafts.

Living standards	Standards are very low; grossly unsanitary conditions prevail at both the public and private levels, and comforts and luxuries are limited to a few elites.	Standards are still quite low but there is some improvement toward the end of the period.
Food and nutrition	Food available to the masses is of poor quality with chronic and occasionally acute shortages. Children and women of fertile years are most affected.	Early improvement in agriculture and crop rotation and increased use of the potato improve nutrition a little. Children and women are still at a nutritional disadvantage.
Health profile		
Mortality pattern	Life expectancy fluctuates around 20 and childhood mortality is very high: one-third of all deaths occur in children from 0–5: 200–300 infant deaths occur per 1,000 births and the neonatal to post-neonatal death ratio is small. Proportionate mortality for 50+ ages is low since few reach that age. Females in the adolescent and reproductive years are at a higher risk of dying than males but at lower risk at older ages. Mortality is somewhat higher in urban than in rural areas.	Mortality remains high but shows signs of declining as fluctuations become less pronounced. Life expectancy increases to mid-twenties and early thirties. Females are still at high risk of dying in the adolescent and fertile years. Infant and childhood mortality are high with small neonatal to post-neonatal ratio; proportionate mortality of the 50+ ages increases somewhat. Urban mortality remains higher than rural.
Disease pattern	Leading causes of death and disease are the epidemic scourges, endemic, parasitic and deficiency diseases, pneumonia–diarrhoea–malnutrition complex in children, and tuberculosis–puerperal–malnutrition complex in females. Manifest famines occur and severe malnutrition underlies disease and death from most other causes.	Leading causes of death and disease are endemic, parasitic and deficiency diseases, epidemic scourges, childhood and maternal complexes. Industrial disease increases. Under-nutrition, though somewhat ameliorated, continues to be important.
Disease examples	(1) Tuberculosis is more virulent in young females, especially in their fertile years. (2) Smallpox is typically a childhood disease. (3) Heart disease rates are low, with high rheumatic to arteriosclerotic ratio. (4) Deficiency disease symptomatology is typical and highly prevalent.	(1) Tuberculosis mortality peaks with industrialisation; it is still more virulent in young females. (2) Smallpox is still chiefly a disease of childhood. (3) Heart disease is still low, with a high rheumatic to arteriosclerotic ratio. (4) Death from starvation is less frequent but typical deficiency diseases still occur.

Table 7.1. (continued)

Transition Profiles	Age of Pestilence and Famine	Age of receding pandemics (early)
Community health profiles	The leading community health problems are epidemics, famine, under-nutrition, childhood disease and maternal death, all aggravated by environmental problems (contaminated water and food, poor housing, insects, rodents) and lack of personal hygiene. There are no medical care systems and few decisive therapies. People have to rely on indigenous healing and witchcraft.	Epidemics, famine, under-nutrition, childhood disease and maternal death are important, environmental problems persist, and industrial health problems emerge. There are no medical care systems and few decisive therapies; hospitals are seen as 'death traps'. People rely on indigenous systems of healing, but personal hygiene and nutrition begin to improve slowly.
	Age of receding pandemics (late)	Age of degenerative and man-made diseases
	Mortality slowly but progressively declines from higher than to lower than 30/1,000. Several decades after mortality declines, fertility starts to decline also. Population growth is explosive for most of this period.	Mortality declines rapidly to below 20/1,000; then the rate of decline slows. Fertility declines to below 20/1,000 (with occasional rises, e.g. the post-Second World War baby boom) and becomes chief pace maker of population growth; fluctuation is by design more than by chance. Population growth is small but persistent.
	The young dependency ratio goes up as the proportion of children in the population increases; there is a slight increase in the old dependency ratio. Improved female survival results in an excess of females. There is continued emigration to colonies, and a substantial increase in rural to urban migration, with concomitant growth of industrial centres.	There is a progressive aging of the population as fertility continues to decline and more people, especially females, survive to middle and old age. The male/female ratio continues to decrease. There is a high and increasing old dependency ratio, especially for women. Residence is increasingly urban, with excessive growth of cities (megapolitanism) and alarming slum formation, environmental pollution, and unwieldy social and political problems.
	'Take-off' to sustained economic growth can often be traced to sharp stimuli such as scientific discovery or political revolution, which galvanize business and labour to reinforce gains in gross, real and per capita income through reinvestment and speculation.	Scientific expertise and applied technology covering the gamut of economic activities produce spiralling growth initially. Then a stage of high mass consumption brings tapered growth as production shifts from producer to consumer goods and services; public welfare and leisure spending increase.

An era of rising expectations touches nearly all segments of society.

Rational–purposive lifestyles prevail; bureaucracy and depersonalisation foster anomic groups.

Extended, large families persist in rural areas; nuclear families prevail increasingly in urban centers. Many women are employed in factories and become more involved in activities outside the home.

Nuclear families and small family size norms become institutionalised. Women are increasingly emancipated from traditional roles and become better educated and more career oriented.

Hygiene and sanitation improve, except in city slums where bad conditions grow worse.

Progressive rises in living conditions are enjoyed by large segments of the population.

Continued improvements in agricultural technology guarantee better availability and quality of food.

People become extremely conscious of nutrition, especially that of children and mothers. There is, however, a tendency to over-nutrition including consumption of rich and high-fat foods, which may increase the risk of heart and metabolic diseases.

There is a considerable change in mortality level and pattern with the recession of pandemics. Life expectancy increases to 30 to 40+. Mortality declines favour children under 15 and women in the fertile years. Infant mortality drops below 150/1,000 births and the neonatal to post-neonatal ratio increases progressively. Proportionate mortality of the 50+ ages increases to close to 50%.

Life expectancy reaches an unprecedented high of 70+ and is about three or more years higher for women than for men. Risks for females of all ages decrease, and maternal mortality declines to a minimum. The age profile shows reductions in childhood mortality, which account for less than 10% of the total deaths, while deaths at 50+ years increase to 70% or more of the total. Infant mortality is less than 25/1,000 and the ratio of neonatal to post-neonatal deaths is large and still increasing.

Pandemics of infection, malnutrition and childhood disease recede; plagues disappear. Cholera sweeps Europe in successive waves before disappearing. Infection remains the leading cause of death, but non-infectious diseases begin to be more significant.

Heart disease, cancer and stroke replace infection as prime killers. Pneumonia, bronchitis, influenza and some viral diseases remain problems. Polio rises, and then tapers off. Scarlet fever starts to disappear.

Table 7.1. (continued)

	Age of receding pandemics (late)	Age of degenerative and man-made diseases
	(1) Tuberculosis declines but there is still a slight excess in young females. (2) Smallpox starts to occur less in children and more in adults due to the vaccination of children. (3) Heart disease increases, and there is a decrease in the rheumatic to arteriosclerotic ratio. (4) Death from starvation is rare, and many deficiency diseases such as scurvy start to disappear.	(1) Tuberculosis is low but persists in slum populations and in older disadvantaged individuals, especially males. (2) Smallpox is rare, and when it does occur, it is a disease of adults. (3) Heart disease is high, with a very low rheumatic to arteriosclerotic ratio. (4) Starvation is rare; pellagra disappears; rickets drops off.
	Epidemics and famines recede; childhood disease and maternal death decrease. Environmental control – e.g. water filtration, refuse pick-up – is started in cities. Health systems develop but are limited in scope. A few decisive therapies and prophylactic measures are devised. The importance of workers' health is recognized. Personal hygiene and nutrition improve.	Morbidity comes to overshadow mortality as an index of health as degenerative and chronic disease problems prevail and mental illness, addiction, accidents, radiation hazards and other pollution problems become more prevalent. More decisive therapies are available, and health systems gradually become oriented to preventive care and case-finding, although rising medical costs become a stubborn health problem.

Source: Adapted from Omran (1971)

of each of these phases. The first is 'The Age of Pestilence and Famine'. Omran characterises this period as one with high, fluctuating mortality (and fertility) rates and where infectious diseases are responsible for the majority of deaths. Early human societies were exposed to a battery of lethal pathogens, viruses and bacteria. Some of these, such as malaria, pinworms and body lice were inherited from primate ancestors and have evolved with us (Armelagos et al. 2005). Although Omran is rather vague about when this period starts, a number of writers argue that the Neolithic revolution brought an explosion in the number, range and impact of infectious diseases encountered by humans (Caspari and Lee 2004; Caspari and Lee 2006; Hill et al. 2007; Harper and Armelagos 2010). With the domestication of animals and development of farming technology, human society became increasingly concentrated in larger settlements.

The reliance on primary food production (agriculture) increased the incidence and the impact of disease. Sedentism, an important feature of agricultural adaptation, conceivably increased parasitic disease spread by contact with human waste ... The domestication of animals provided a steady supply of vectors and greater exposure to zoonotic diseases. The zoonotic infections most likely increased because of domesticated animals, such as goats, sheep, cattle, pigs, and fowl, as well as the unwanted domestic animals such as rodents and sparrows.

(Armelagos *et al.* 1996: 2–3)

Fitzpatrick (2008) identifies four types of diseases that were responsible for the major causes of death during this period; (i) airborne diseases, such as TB and influenza; (ii) waterborne diseases, like cholera, giardia, typhoid and botulism; (iii) food-borne diseases, like dysentery and; (iv) vector-borne diseases, such as the Black Death. Ironically, given improvements in farming, famine is also a main cause of death during this period.

Omran's second stage is 'The Age of Receding Pandemics'. As the name suggests, during this phase infectious diseases steadily give way to non-communicable diseases as the main cause of death. Consequently, mortality rates decline and population growth accelerates. Life expectancy also increases and becomes more stable. Again Omran is rather vague on the historical periodisation of this transition. However he does divide this stage into its early and late phases. The early phase could well describe the Agricultural Revolution that occurred in Britain and Europe in the 1700s, which saw the introduction of new farming methods and technologies, such as the seed-drill and iron plough (Overton, 2002). This led to an increase in both the quantity and quality of food available. The later phase appears to correspond to the early stages of the (first) Industrial Revolution. This saw the growth of small-scale factory production, in cottage industries and the putting-out system, driven by a number of technological advances such as the spinning jenny. Life expectancy and populations continued to increase. However, infectious diseases, like TB, remained major killers. But now cardiovascular diseases become more prominent, especially amongst the richer sections of society.

Omran's final stage is 'The Age of Degenerative and Man-Made Diseases'. Following the transition to this phase infectious diseases have been all but eliminated as causes of death. In their place chronic diseases, such as CVD, and lifestyle illnesses, such as alcoholism, have become the major causes of mortality. As a result mortality and fertility rates decline and then level off, and population growth slows dramatically. This is the stage about which Omran is the most clear. He suggests that these changes began around the middle of the nineteenth century and gives data from a number of countries from the late 1880s onwards to illustrate his argument. The socio-economic correlates of this transition are clearly linked to advanced forms of capitalism. He identifies the increasingly technological nature of the production process and the growth of the tertiary sector as the economic characteristics of this stage. According to his model these bring with them improvements in material living standards and greater gender equality.

From Table 7.1 one can see that in the ETT there is a clear connection between socio-economic change and the main causes of death in any given society. However, and this is key for our argument, Omran argues that, although the relationship is complex, it is socio-economic change that drives epidemiological change. In line with his fourth proposition he argues that

> it is relatively certain that, with the possible exception of smallpox, the recession of plague and many other pandemics in Europe was in no way related to the progress of science ... The reduction of mortality in Europe and most western countries during the nineteenth century, as described by the classical model of the epidemiologic transition, was determined primarily through ecobiologic and socioeconomic factors.
>
> (Omran 1971: 520)

This is a crucial aspect of ETT and separates it from other, more demographically or technologically determinist, approaches. However it also invites a host of sociological questions about the nature and pace of these socioeconomic changes.

Omran addresses these in his fifth proposition by positing three models of the epidemiological transition. These are the classical or Western model, the accelerated model and the contemporary or delayed model. Clearly the model that he describes in some detail in Table 7.1 represents a classic trajectory through the various stages. Countries like the US and the UK are held up as examples of this model with a relatively long first and second stage and the early onset of the third stage of the epidemiological transition. As already noted these stages map on to a fairly standard, although not unproblematic, account of the modernisation of these countries. As these countries became successively more industrialised and urbanised the diseases that had been the scourge of earlier periods on history were largely eradicated. This argument was neither novel nor unique. (McKeown 1976; McKeown *et al.* 1972) had made similar observations on the effects of the improved standard of living, better sanitation and diet on the health of populations following industrialisation. As the name suggests, in the accelerated model a country passes through the same stages but the transition from the age of receding pandemics to the age of degenerative diseases takes place in a much more concentrated time period. Japan is portrayed as an example of the accelerated model. However, he is rather vague about why this transition was so rapid in these countries and, reflecting Weisz and Olszynko-Gryn's (2010) arguments, he is more focused on the decline in fertility than the shift in the causes of death.

> [T]he drop in mortality in the twentieth century, which was determined by sanitary and medical advances as well as by general social improvements. In these countries, national and individual aspirations favored a controlled rate of population increase and provided the intense motivation needed to lower fertility in a relatively short period of time.
>
> (Omran 1971: 535)

Finally the delayed model 'describes the relatively recent and yet-to-be-completed transition of most developing countries'. These countries have begun to experience declines in mortality but fertility rates remain high. He argues that contrary to the classical model, public health and 'imported, internationally sponsored medical package[s]' have been chiefly responsible for the fall in mortality rates. Again, however, Omran is quiet about why the epidemiological transition in these countries has been delayed. Therefore, although Omran cannot be accused of ignoring international variations in the pace and nature of this transition, he does not give an adequate explanation as to why certain countries depart from the classical model and why, amongst that group, some are able to 'catch up' with the West while others have a delayed trajectory. This is a serious weakness in his theory and prevents it from achieving its potential to help reduce the amount of preventable deaths around the world.

Empirically ETT is supported by a range of historical data from the UK (Mooney 2007) and France (Coste et al. 2006) as well as more recent data from countries in Europe (Spijker and Llorens 2009), Asia (Joshi et al. 2006; Ahsan Karar et al. 2009; Chan et al. 2009; Manderson and Naemiratch 2010), Latin America (Young 1994; Albala et al. 2002; Fraser 2006) and the developing world more generally (Shen and Williamson 2001; Salomon and Murray 2002; Shandra et al. 2004; Houweling et al. 2005; Miranda et al. 2008; Stuckler 2008; Gaziano 2010; Gaziano et al. 2010; Gersh et al. 2010; Lloyd-Sherlock 2010).

However Omran has also attracted a good deal of criticism. It has been argued that he overstated the pace and extent of the decline of infectious diseases in the developed world (Condrau and Worboys 2007; Lussier et al. 2008). There is another family of critiques that, whilst generally supportive of the basic premise of the ETT, has sought to adapt or extend Omran's taxonomy by proposing new stages. There are a number of competitors for a fourth stage of the epidemiological transition. Some have argued that contrary to Omran's original prediction life expectancy has not levelled off but has continued to fall, heralding a new stage of 'delayed degenerative disease' in many of the advanced industrial countries (Olshansky and Ault 1986; Rogers and Hackenberg 1987). Alternatively a number of writers have argued that the fourth stage is characterised by the persistence or even re-emergence of infectious diseases alongside chronic illnesses, which has resulted in a 'double burden' of disease in many developing countries (Armelagos et al. 1996; Caselli et al. 2002; Greger 2007; Hill et al. 2007; Stevens et al. 2008; Stratton et al. 2008; Huicho et al. 2009).

Whilst these observations are important and have helped to improve the ETT, they too suffer from the same methodologically nationalist focus that characterises the original model. As has already been noted Omran explicitly weds his theory of epidemiological transition to modernisation theory. But, as Shen and Williamson (2001: 258) argue:

> Modernization/free trade theory was originally formulated on the basis of historical developments in Western industrial countries, but many theorists have been critical of efforts to generalize this perspective to the [less developed

countries] today. Some critics claim that modernization/free trade theory fails both to describe the current Third World reality or to interpret its future path ... it does not give adequate attention to inequality within societies, including gender inequality or to structural relations between the core and non-core countries in the world economy.

From a WST perspective such an approach makes two key, and erroneous, assumptions. First, that what happened in the West will inevitably happen in every other country. Second, that each nation is an independent actor free from interference. A key argument from WST is that countries in the developing world are not simply earlier versions of countries in the developed world. This is because instead of seeing individual countries as separate units, each following a linear trajectory, states form part of an interconnected whole. They are parts of a system and their development, or under-development, is deeply connected to their place in this system. Therefore a WST approach allows us to correct the state-centrism of the ETT and opens up two key areas of research. First how, today and in the past, infectious diseases might be transmitted between states. Second how world-system dynamics prevent societies from achieving socio-economic conditions necessary to pass through the successive epidemiological transitions.

World systems theory

At its base

> a world-system is a social system, one that has boundaries, structures, member groups, rules of legitimation, and coherence. Its life is made up of the conflicting forces which hold it together by tension and tear it apart as each group seeks eternally to remould it to its advantage. It has the characteristics of an organism, in that it has a lifespan over which its characteristics change in some respects and remain stable in others ... Life within it is largely self-contained, and the dynamics of its development are largely internal.
>
> (Wallerstein 1974: 347)

Immanuel Wallerstein defines the world-system as

> a system that is a world and which can be, most often has been, located in an area less than the entire globe. World-systems analysis argues that the units of social reality within which we operate, whose rules constrain us, are for the most part such world-systems (other than the now extinct, small mini-systems that once existed on the earth). World-system analysis argues that there have been thus far only two varieties of world-systems: world-economies and world-empires. A world-empire (examples, the Roman Empire, Han China) are large bureaucratic structures with a single political center and an axial

division of labor, but multiple cultures. A world-economy is a large axial division of labor with multiple political centers and multiple cultures.

(Wallerstein 2004: 98)

For Wallerstein the movement to a capitalist world economy was a crucial transition. He saw the emergence of the capitalist world-system as Eurocentric, with the inevitable positioning of peripheral areas as sources of labour power in the production of commodities for core markets. Wallerstein's work made a break with modernisation theory and many of the principles of the then fashionable development theory. The latter was really premised on the notion that 'poor', 'third world' countries could develop successfully if they adopted US and European approaches, and presumably also adopt a US and European disease profile. Wallerstein demonstrates the inadequacy of the modernisation premises, and in common with dependency theorists and many others showed that much of the inequality in the world and the consequent issues for disease is structural.

With this transition the world was effectively split into three zones or regions. These were the core, semi-periphery and periphery. In this schema countries in the core were the developed, industrialised economies, and those in the periphery are the 'underdeveloped' economies, typically those reliant on the export of raw materials to the core. Thus the world system operates as a set of mechanisms that redistributes resources from the periphery to the core. These classifications may best be seen as ideal types. Nonetheless core countries could be expected to exhibit some common features. They would:

- be the most economically diversified, wealthy and powerful countries;
- have a strong central government, a strong state and a sufficient tax base so these state institutions can provide infrastructure for a strong economy;
- be highly industrialised and produce manufactured goods rather than raw materials for export;
- increasingly tend to specialise in information, finance and service industries;
- be at the forefront of new technologies and new industries;
- have a strong bourgeoisie and an organised working class;
- have significant means of influence over nations in the (semi)periphery and themselves be relatively independent of outside control.

Conversely countries in the periphery have a weak industrial base and tend to depend on a small number of commodities, largely primary goods and/or raw materials. They tend to have weak, corrupt governments with disarticulated state structures. They have a large informal and agricultural workforce. They tend to have low education and literacy rates in the population. They also have high levels of inequality with the wealth concentrated amongst a small elite. Finally, and most importantly, they are dominated, economically, politically and militarily, by the core countries.

How then does WST match against the epidemiological transition, and how do possibly different examples of transition interrelate? To answer such a question we need to be prepared to examine and compare different world-systems. Comparative world-system approaches start from the point where sedentary human groups were first identified on the planet, about twelve thousand years ago. The definition of world-systems for comparative research changes to:

> Intersocietal networks in which the interactions (e.g. trade, warfare, intermarriage, information) are important for the reproduction of the internal structures of the composite units and importantly affect changes that occur in these local structures.
>
> (Chase-Dunn and Hall 1996: 404)

The term 'composite units' means more than 'society'; the latter term commonly suggests a clearly bounded social group. World-systems, however, have to be conceived as social structures based on biological and ecological substrata that include different cultural groupings and polities. They are distinct from ecological and biological systems. The first world-systems started with sedentarism and the active combination of sedentary 'villages' and 'diversified foragers'. From this emerged territorialism and the beginning of collective property and boundary maintenance between groups. Foraging and sedentary activity involved the depletion of natural resources and their over-exploitation. Of course the impact of disease is important here and disease patterns can be understood as existing in and through patterns of interaction between human groupings created in and through different systems. The definition used here from Chase-Dunn and Hall retains Wallerstein's emphasis on system but directs our attention less to the emergence of a single system and more to the ways in which different networks operate within world-systems. Where Wallerstein sought to capture this through terms such as mini-system, empire and economy, with a central focus on the move to a capitalist world-economy and its subsequent development, we will follow Chase-Dunn and Hall and review interlinking systems that we feel enable better linkages with epidemiological transitions. We do so by reviewing the analytic categories proposed by Chase-Dunn and Hall.

How world-systems are constructed

Inevitably many world-systems will be small, particularly in the case of sedentary and nomadic societies. Interactions are with immediate neighbours rather than more widespread. Transportation systems and information flow would be fairly restricted at this point in time. However, we can identify features such as production, communication, warfare, alliances and trade found in early world-systems (see Chew (2005) for examples). Some developments and changes within systems will be endogenous while others will not. An exogenous impact that might change a system would include, following Chase-Dunn and Hall (1996), a parasite that attacks a population without immunity and depletes the population drastically. While this is certainly a disease impact it is not a world-system effect unless two or more areas are linked through some of the systemic networks. When the parasitic or similar assault, such as the 'black death' where fleas were carried by rats, affects countries bound by trade then we can refer to this as a world-system disease effect. Trade relations are regularised and the disease spread also becomes regularised. The effects of influenza, brought to parts of South America and the Caribbean by Spanish and Portuguese in the sixteenth century, are also a systemic feature because of the regularised exploitative relations of the parts within a European world-system. The constituents of world-systems include boundaries created by:

- bulk goods exchange network (BGN);
- prestige goods exchange network (PGN);
- political/military exchange network (PMN);
- information exchange network (IN).

The bulk goods network for trade links were to become core and peripheries in the early capitalist world-economy and world-system. But a bulk trade network will be a relatively small interregional network because of the costs involved in transportation. It may well also include political agreements and commercial arrangements. These may form an independent network and a complex set of arrangements may link more than one bulk goods network. In the fifteenth and sixteenth centuries bulk goods such as timber and wool linked different parts of Europe through a political exchange network that also supported the carrying of a prestige goods network based on gold and silver bullion from the Americas.

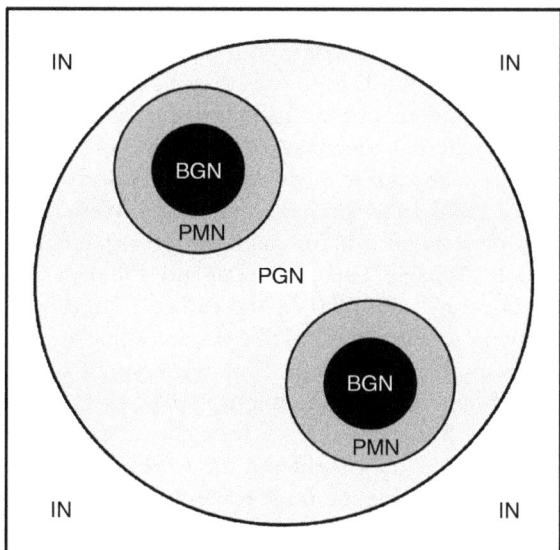

Figure 7.1 Spatial boundaries of world-system networks

The four networks are of different sizes. Following Chase-Dunn and Hall (1996; 1997), Figure 7.1 shows how the networks might be linked.

Here the information exchange network is presented as outside the other networks. Exchange of goods involves exchange of information but sometimes the goods exchange is greater than the amount of information involved. Thus bulk or prestige objects may be passed on from one partner to another but the information does not get passed on in the same way. Some pieces of information may stick at certain points and some may be seen as redundant. This has implications for how diseases are described, evaluated and explained. Thus the information network for disease may be specialised, e.g. professionals evaluating treatment programmes, but it may only achieve impact through the prestige networks available, thus ensuring potential distributors of vaccines are approached as holders of prestige connections. Our point is that different system configurations are possible, and each may constitute a world-system as defined above.

Refining the categories of analysis

In addition to the categories given above we need to introduce what Wallerstein termed 'the external zone':

> from the point of view of the capitalist world-economy, an external arena was a zone from which the capitalist world-economy wanted goods but which was resistant (perhaps culturally) to importing manufactured goods in return and strong enough politically to maintain its preferences.
>
> (Wallerstein 1989: 167)

Such zones may not form an immediate part of the capitalist world-system but they provide a locus for disease parasites, both waterborne and airborne, that can enter established world systems. The point is that their place within world-system activity would not be random but could follow particular contours. Thus one possibility might be an external zone that either initiates or becomes involved in a disease transmission even though it is external to the world-system. Abu-Lughod (1989) traces the Black Death in its reach from the east to Western Europe by largely accepting McNeill's presentation. If we combine the arguments of both we find the four disease pools (McNeill 1976; Abu-Lughod 1989) map onto the world-systems of the periods from 1250–1350 CE and earlier. Both show that the warring invasions and settlements spread infectious diseases according to a pattern of transfer when people had not built up immunity. The disease-pool approach maps onto world-system developments and as one might expect an external zone, such as that of the Slav peoples from 400–900 CE lying in the external zone, remained free of the infectious diseases until it entered the world-system.

These peoples were not outside the trade routes but they were not incorporated into the empire. In terms of human destruction McNeill notes they avoided the fate of the urban peasantries of the Mediterranean south and elsewhere in the empire. They also avoided the microparasitic transmissions suffered in the empire, which meant their population increased. When they expanded into Western Europe and further west they became part of the microparasitic transmission chain, suffering severe population loss at first and then a subsequent balancing as immunity was built up.

The external zone does not act as a neutral party in epidemiological terms. It would appear to be that as external zones are incorporated, usually into the periphery, so they face severe illness and depredation initially. However, as the number of external zones has decreased, now reaching a point where there may be no such zones at all within a capitalist system, the epidemiological pattern may change.

Dependency and disease

The foregoing gives us a much more integrated, systemic, framework for understanding how infectious diseases may have been spread in the past and what might contribute to their re-emergence today. However the WST approach also raises another, perhaps more current, issue of the impact of core–periphery relations on the epidemiological transition. If we take Omran's fourth proposition to be true, that societies need to achieve certain levels of socio-economic development in order to pass through successive stages of the epidemiological transition, then world-system dynamics, which keep peripheral countries in a state of dependency, ought to also impact on the health of the population in these countries.

In order to test this argument it is necessary to look at the impact of external factors, rather than internal factors, such as GDP or urbanisation, on the causes of death in a population. As noted earlier, to the best of knowledge, no one has explicitly tried to bring WST and ETT together before. However, similar issues have been explored elsewhere, which we aim to build on. A number of studies have examined the detrimental effects of trade dependency on overall mortality rates (Dixon 1984; London and Williams 1990; Ragin and Bradshaw 1992). More recently Shen and Williamson (2001) have looked at the effects of various forms of dependency on infant mortality. Although both of these are key indicators of ETT none of these studies have looked directly at the main indictor, the cause of death. However they do suggest which indicators of dependency might be used. Shen and Williamson (2001) employ three measures of dependency: trade dependency, debt dependency and investment dependency. However, we have chosen to look only at the first of these as we feel the measure of investment dependency (FDI stock) is inadequate. This is because, unlike the trade dependency measure, it does not give an indication of the relative sectoral concentration, for example in the clothing industry, of FDI. Also data on external debt were only available on the World Bank website for developing countries and therefore lacked sufficient variation for these analyses.

Trade dependency is measured using a commodity concentration index[1] (CCI) taken from the World Trade Organisation (WTO). This is a measure of how diversified a country's exports are on a scale of 0 to 1. A score of 1 would mean that a country's exports are solely dependent on one commodity, such as oil or wheat. The more reliant a country is on a narrow export base then the more vulnerable it is to vagaries of the world market. If the world price for a commodity that makes up the majority of a country's exports falls rapidly then this will have a much more dramatic effect than if this was one of hundreds of commodities all of which were roughly of equal importance (Soutar 1977; Tegene 1990; Savvides and Mohtadi 1991).

In the following analyses we aim to update the previous studies on all-cause and infant mortality in relation to trade dependency as well as extending these analyses to look at the proportion of deaths due to communicable, maternal, perinatal and nutritional diseases. All these data were taken from the World Health Organisation (WHO) website. However the most recent data on cause of death were for 2004.

Figure 7.2 shows that even in 2008 there is a positive, albeit moderate, relationship ($r = .334$) between the degree to which a country is dependent on a relatively narrow range of exports and the level of overall mortality in the population. For example Angola has a mortality rate of 421/100,000 and is highly reliant on crude oil, which makes up over 90 per cent of its exports (CIA World Factbook, 2008). However there are a number of countries that seem to go against the trend. Of particular interest is Zimbabwe, which has a relatively diversified export base (CCI) but has the highest mortality rate ([772/100],000). However it is worth remembering that in 2008 Zimbabwe suffered one of a number of recent devastating outbreaks of cholera (http://www.who.int/csr/don/2008_12_02/en/index.html, accessed 9 December 2011). Figure 7.3 shows a similar, somewhat stronger, relationship ($r = .412$) for mortality rates amongst

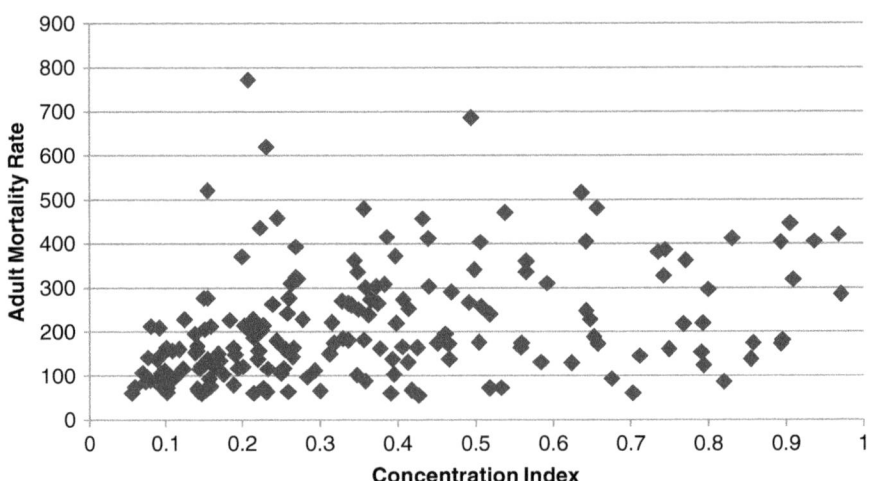

Figure 7.2 Adult mortality rate (per 100,000) by export concentration index: 2008
Source: WHO; WTO

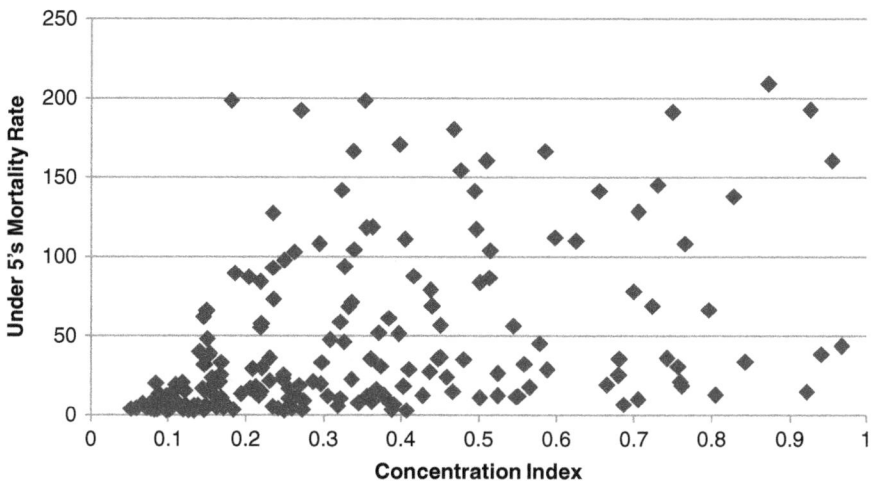

Figure 7.3 Under fives mortality rate (per 100,000) by export concentration index: 2009
Source: World Bank; WTO

under fives. The more restricted a country's export base the higher the rate of infant mortality. Both these findings are generally in line with those found in previous studies and strongly suggest that countries that are in a weaker global trade position, which is a key indicator of occupying a peripheral position in the world system, continue to suffer from mortality rates indicative of Omran's age of infectious diseases and pandemics. Turning, then, to the key issue of the cause of death, Figure 7.3 shows a strong relationship between the CCI and proportion deaths attributable to communicable, maternal, perinatal and nutritional conditions ($r = .448$).

West Africa: the impact of the world system on disease and death

These analyses demonstrate a need for the ETT to move beyond its state centricism. This is reinforced if one considers change over time in specific regions of the world. Our suggestions here are speculative at present and need further development. We draw on ideas of how a combination of the two traditions might be taken forward with a focus on West Africa. We have chosen West Africa because it is a region with anticipated high population growth (Cour and Snvech 1998; UN-Habitat 2003; Davis 2006) and consequently an important reflector of disease tendencies.

Our interest here is on how the region might appear taking the map in Figure 7.1 and recasting it at different historical moments. Figure 7.1 is a generic map and any location will have a specific patterning at different times. Our interest lies in considering how the pattern of goods distribution as set out in Figure 7.1 would be drawn at different historical periods and what implications, if any, this holds for ETT.

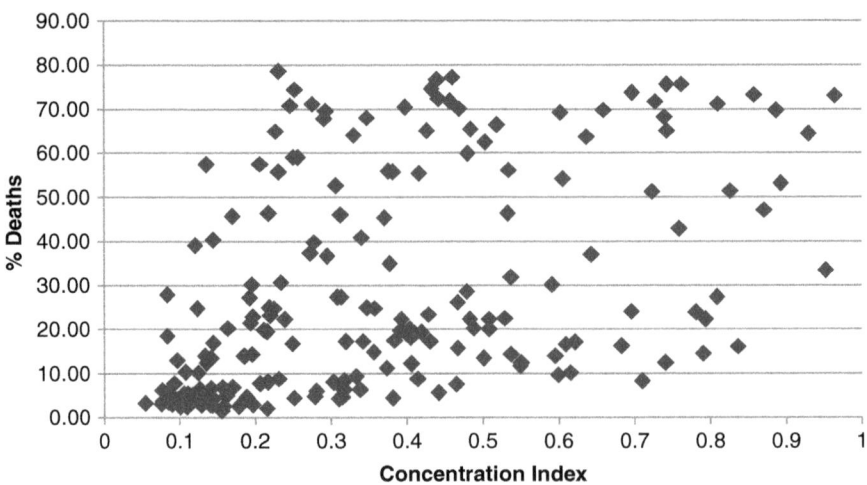

Figure 7.4 Proportion of deaths due to communicable, maternal, perinatal and nutritional conditions by export concentration index: 2004
Source: WHO; WTO

Summarising important histories of the West African region (Dike 1956; Crowder 1966; Crowder 1968; Hopkins 1977), we can distinguish a number of distinctive periods: an extensive period from BCE that goes on to include the major African empires, the period of European discovery and the beginnings of European control (1500–1700), the period of the slave trade (1700–1800s), the colonial period lasting up to decolonisation (1860–1960s), and the most recent period (1960s onwards). Our suggestion is that there will be differences in both the size of the segments (bulk goods trade, prestige goods trade, political and military networks and the resulting information networks). The factors that influence such changes include of course the forms of trade, political and social relations in place that will change as the region is first incorporated as an external zone and peripheralised. What WST leaves out is an account of the changing patterns of disease, instead seeing disease as an outcome of people movements. We have suggested it is more complex than that.

At the risk of simplification we posit that in the long period from BCE until the end of the kingdoms in the sixteenth century trade in bulk goods and prestige goods was largely in balance. The proportion of each to the other was roughly proportionate over this long time period. This was in part because 'fly free' lines (Lambrecht 1964; Steverding 2008) were found and retained so trade took on a regular pattern. The region was not entirely self-contained because the trade in salt, slaves and other goods across the Sahara brought people into contact with a number of disease pools. However, once European exploration occurred from the fifteenth century onwards the information aspect of the system changed, which then acted upon the then world-system leading to changes in goods traded.

As European supercargoes became established, developing trade in palm oil from the sixteenth century, so new factors came into play (Okonta and Douglas 2003). In brief, bulk goods trade declined and prestige goods trade increased leading to far greater movement of peoples. This was then extended through the slave trade and the peripheralisation of West Africa in the European world-system. The slave trade itself led to the rise of sleeping sickness caused by the tsetse fly. The West African populations had largely achieved immunity against the fly but the incursion of chained slaves forcibly marched to the slave ports led to new outbreaks. The colonial period saw the beginning of a tendency that has increased much faster since – movement of peoples from the northern part of the region to the cities of the south. Lagos is one of the fastest growing cities in Africa. This movement is part trade related and it leads to the rise of diseases associated with poor sanitation and lack of clean water supplies. As Steverding (2008: 5) notes in relation to the Congo:

> Other factors that affected the epidemiology of sleeping sickness in the first half of the last century are the socio-economic conditions created during the colonisation of Africa. An excellent example of this is the sleeping sickness epidemic in the north-central Uele district of the former Belgian Congo, now known as the Democratic Republic of Congo. Colonisation of this region in the first decade of the 19th century was protracted and brutal. Large numbers of people were displaced and many of them experienced famine. This created an ideal environment for spreading the disease and sleeping sickness became increasingly entrenched and epidemic in this region over the next 15 years. It was not until the mid 1920s that medical services were introduced in the Uele district by the colonial powers.

The region has also been plagued by intermittent but persistent warfare, such as the Nigerian Civil War of 1967–70. This increase in political–military networks since decolonisation has not only led to some 13 million deaths through starvation and warfare, but the conflict also increased the attractiveness of the Niger Delta to the government. The development of the oil-refining industry is the most obvious illustration of this. In terms of our world-system model Nigeria in particular has reverted from a mixed export provider of bulk goods to reliance on a single export – oil (Nnadozie 1995). Much of the profit has been drained off and the Delta region is significantly poorer than the rest of the country. The rise in cancers and diarrhoeal illnesses that claim many lives in this area have been exacerbated by the activities of the private militias hired by the oil companies. Such diseases were certainly less common before the expansion of the oil refineries. The question of whether oil refining is causing a rise in disease is not our question here. Rather, our purpose is to indicate that a significant trade pattern in one commodity has emerged alongside a shift in disease types. The issue here is the type of position West Africa plays in the largely single world-system found today. The OECD and WHO data given above show that it is in a different position from that of the OECD countries. Attributing this to limited modernisation or development is misleading. A more compelling explanation would involve tracking the impacts of major companies on the West Africa region, including measures of the effects of clean-up operations from toxic wastes, and the impacts on health of export zones used to handle toxic materials. Without pre-empting what data would show we can suggest that an examination of the changing shape of the world-system at different historical times will reflect changes in epidemiology and lead to a fruitful combination of two theoretical traditions.

Conclusion

In conclusion we hope to have shown the benefit of the bringing together of ETT and WST for researchers from both fields. Our aim has not been to refute or reject ETT. We feel that this has been an important contribution to our understanding of population health and a corrective to the demographically or biologically deterministic alternatives. As noted earlier there is plenty of evidence to support Omran's premise and some of the criticisms are based on misrepresentations of the model. However we feel that it is important to challenge its state-centricism and this provided us with an ideal vehicle to explore the potential utility of adopting a WST approach. Thus we have focused on ETT because of its clear 'complementarity' with some of the principle components of the WST. They both share a focus on populations and modernisation theory as a common reference point. We certainly feel that bringing these two theories together opens up a host of potential research areas. For example it would be possible to revisit the reasons for transitions in history and look at the existence of trade networks and military and political alliances on the development of systems, and how these impact upon mortality and fertility profiles. On a macro-level more sophisticated statistical models could be built to explore the impact of trade dependency alongside other indicators, such as political and military power relations, on mortality profiles. Alternatively, or in addition, more micro-level analyses could focus on specific regions, such as the Niger Delta. In this regard the more recent work on what is called 'epidemiological polarization' (Frenk et al. 1989; Frenk et al. 1991) raises some important issues. Writers such as Dummer and Cook (2008) and Bobadilla and de Possas (1992) and Huynen and colleagues (2005) have all argued that a number of developing countries are experiencing this polarisation as urban, metropolitan centres pass into the third phase, leaving the rural hinterlands behind in the age of pandemics and infectious diseases. Such observations lend themselves to analyses through a WST approach with its focus less on states but rather, as Chase-Dunn and Hall (1996) note, on networks.

However the possibilities offered by incorporating a WST approach to medical sociology and/or social epidemiology need not be restricted to ETT. A number of the features of WST share many common concerns with those found in other areas of health research. As Wallerstein notes countries in the periphery tend to be more iniquitous, with colonial or comprador elites dominating resources. This invites further exploration in line with the work already done by writers such as Wilkinson (2001; 2005; 2009) on the effects of inequalities on health. Another possibility might be to look at the impact of world system dynamics on the (dis)organisation of welfare states. A key feature of the WST model is that states in the periphery are weak and often highly corrupt. Such observations echo recent analyses on different types of insecurity and welfare regimes in the developing world (Gough *et al.* 2008). In short we feel that many different areas of sociological research in and around aspects of health might benefit from further engagement with the work of Wallerstein and the wider WST approach.

Note

1 Concentration index, also named Herfindahl-Hirschmann index, is a measure of the degree of market concentration. It has been normalized to obtain values ranking from 0 to 1 (maximum concentration), according to the following formula:

$$H_j = \frac{\sqrt{\sum_{i=1}^{n} \left(\frac{x_i}{X}\right)^2} - \sqrt{1=n}}{1 - \sqrt{1=n}}$$

where Hj = country or country group index
xi = value of exports of product i

$$X = \sum_{i=1}^{n} x_i$$

and n = number of products (SITC Revision 3 at 3-digit group level)

References

Abu-Lughod, J. (1989). *Before European Hegemony: The World System A.D. 1250–1350*. Oxford: Oxford University Press.
Ahsan Karar, Z., Alam, N. and Streatfield, P. (2009). 'Epidemiological transition in rural Bangladesh, 1986–2006'. *Global health action* 2.
Albala, C., Vio, F. Kain, J. and Uauy, R. (2002). 'Nutrition transition in Chile: determinants and consequences'. *Public Health Nutrition* 5(1a): 123–28.
Armelagos, G. J., Barnes, K. C. and Lin, J. (1996). 'Disease in Human Evolution: The Re-Emergence of Infectious Disease in the Third Epidemiological Transition'. *National Museum of Natural History Bulletin for Teachers* 18: 1–6.
Armelagos, G. J., Brown, P. J. and Turnev, B. (2005). 'Evolutionary, historical and political economic perspectives on health and disease'. *Social Science* 65.
Bobadilla, J. L. and Possas, C. de A. (1992). How the epidemiological transition affects health policy isues in three Latin American countries, Washington, D.C: The World Bank.
Braudel, F. (1993). *A History of Civilizations*. London: Penguin.
——(2002a). *The perspective of the world. Civilization and capitalism 15th–18th century. Volume 1*. London: Orion House.
——(2002b). *The structures of everyday life. Civilization and capitalism 15th–18th century. Volume 2*. London: Orion House.
——(2002c). *The wheels of commerce. Civilization and capitalism 15th–18th century. Volume 3*. London: Orion House.
Caselli, G., Mesle, F. et al. (2002). 'Epidemiologic transition theory exceptions'. *Genus* 58: 9–52.

Caspari, R. and Lee, S.-H. (2004). 'Older age becomes common late in human evolution'. *Proceedings of the National Academy of Sciences of the United States of America* 101(30): 10895–900.
——(2006). 'Is human longevity a consequence of cultural change or modern biology?' *American Journal of Physical Anthropology* 129(4): 512–17.
Chan, J. C. N., Malik, V. Jia, W. Kadowaki, T., Yajnik, C. and Yoon, K.-H. (2009). 'Diabetes in Asia'. *JAMA: The Journal of the American Medical Association* 301(20): 2129–40.
Chase-Dunn, C. and Hall, T. (1996). 'Ecological Degradation and the Evolution of World-Systems'. *Journal of World-Systems Research* 3: 403–31.
——(1997). *Rise and Demise: Comparing World-Systems*. Boulder, CO: Westview Press.
Chew, S. C. (2005). 'From Harappa to Mesopotamia and Egypt to Mycenae: Dark Ages, Political-Economic Declines, and Environmental/Climatic Changes 2200 B.C.-700 B.C'. *The Historical Evolution of World-Systems*. C. Chase-Dunn and E. N. Anderson (eds). Basingstoke: Palgrave Macmillan: 52–74.
CIA (2008) *The World Factbook 2008*. Washington, D.C: US Executive Office of the President.
Condrau, F. and Worboys M. (2007). 'Second opinions: Epidemics and infections in nineteenth-century Britain'. *Social History of Medicine* 20(1): 147–58.
Cook, I. G. and Dummer, T. J. B. (2004). 'Changing health in China: re-evaluating the epidemiological transition model'. *Health policy (Amsterdam, Netherlands)* 67(3): 329–43.
Cour, J-M. and Snvech, S. (Eds) (1998) *Preparing for the Future: A Vision of West Africa in the Year 2020*. Paris: OECD.
Coste, J., Bernardin, E. Jougla, E. (2006). 'Patterns of mortality and their changes in France (1968–99): insights into the structure of diseases leading to death and epidemiological transition in an industrialised country'. *Journal of Epidemiology and Community Health* 60(11): 945–55.
Crowder, M. (1966). *The story of Nigeria*. London: Faber and Faber.
——(1968). *West Africa under colonial rule*. London: Northwestern University Press.
Davis, M. (2006) *Planet of Slums*. London: Verso.
Dike, K. O. (1956). *Trade and politics in the Niger Delta, 1830–1885: an introduction to the economic and political history of Nigeria*. Oxford: Oxford University Press.
Dixon, W. J. (1984). 'Trade concentration, economic growth, and the provision of basic human needs'. *Social Science Quarterly* 65(3): 761–74.
Dummer, T. J. B. and Cook, I. G. (2008). 'Health in China and India: A cross-country comparison in a context of rapid globalisation'. *Social Science 605*.
Fitzpatrick, R. (2008). 'Society and Changing Patterns of Disease'. G. Scambler (ed.). *Sociology as applied to medicine*, Saunders/Elsevier: 3–18.
Fraser, B. (2006). 'Peru's epidemiological transition'. *Lancet* 367(9528): 2049–50.
Frenk, J., Bobadilla, J. L. Sepuúlveda, J. and Cervantes, M. (1989). 'Health transition in middle-income countries: new challenges for health care'. *Health Policy and Planning* 4(1): 29–39.
Frenk, J., Frejka, T. Prasartkul, P., Porapakkham, Y., Lim, S. and Lopez, A. (1991). 'The epidemiologic transition in Latin America'. *Boletín de la Oficina Sanitaria Panamericana/Pan American Health Organization* 111: 485–96.
Gaziano, J. M. (2010). 'Fifth Phase of the Epidemiologic Transition The Age of Obesity and Inactivity'. *Jama-Journal of the American Medical Association* 303(3): 275–76.
Gaziano, T. A., Bitton, A. et al. (2010). 'Growing Epidemic of Coronary Heart Disease in Low- and Middle-Income Countries'. *Current Problems in Cardiology* 35(2): 72–115.
Gersh, B. J., K. Sliwa, et al. (2010). 'Novel therapeutic concepts – The epidemic of cardiovascular disease in the developing world: global implications'. *European Heart Journal* 31(6): 642–48B.
Gough, I., Wood, G. et al. (2008). *Insecurity and Welfare Regimes in Asia, Africa and Latin America*. Cambridge: Cambridge University Press.

Greger, M. (2007). 'The human/animal interface: Emergence and resurgence of zoonotic infectious diseases'. *Critical Reviews in Microbiology* 33(4): 243–99.
Harper, K. and Armelagos, G. (2010). 'The Changing Disease-Scape in the Third Epidemiological Transition'. *International Journal of Environmental Research and Public Health* 7(2): 675–97.
Hill, K., Hurtado, A. M. et al. (2007). 'High adult mortality among Hiwi hunter-gatherers: Implications for human evolution'. *Journal of Human Evolution* 52(4): 443–54.
Hill, K., Vapattanawong, P. et al. (2007). 'Epidemiologic transition interrupted: a reassessment of mortality trends in Thailand, 1980–2000'. *International Journal of Epidemiology* 36(2): 374–84.
Hopkins, A. G. (1977). *An economic history of West Africa*. London: Longman.
Houweling, T. A. J., Caspar, A. E. K. Looman, W. and Mackenbach, J. (2005). 'Determinants of under-5 mortality among the poor and the rich: a cross-national analysis of 43 developing countries'. *International Journal of Epidemiology* 34(6): 1257–65.
Huicho, L., Trelles, M. Gonzales, F. Mendoza, W. and Miranda, J. (2009). 'Mortality profiles in a country facing epidemiological transition: An analysis of registered data'. *Bmc Public Health* 9: 47–59.
Huynen, M., Vollebregt, L. Martens, P. and Benavides, B. (2005). 'The epidemiologic transition in Peru'. *Pan American Journal of Public Health* 17: 51–59.
Joshi, R., Cardona, M. et al. (2006). 'Chronic diseases now a leading cause of death in rural India – mortality data from the Andhra Pradesh Rural Health Initiative.' *International Journal of Epidemiology* 35(6): 1522–29.
Lambrecht, F. L. (1964). 'Aspects of Evolution and Ecology of Tsetse Flies and Trypanosomiasis in Prehistoric African Environment'. *The Journal of African History* 5: 1–24.
Lloyd-Sherlock, P. (2010). 'Stroke in Developing Countries: Epidemiology, Impact and Policy Implications'. *Development Policy Review* 28(6): 693–709.
London, B. and Williams, B. A. (1990). 'National Politics, International Dependency, and Basic Needs Provision – A Cross-National Analysis'. *Social Forces* 69(2): 565–84.
Lussier, M. H., Bourbeau, R. and Choiniever. R. (2008). 'Does the recent evolution of Canadian mortality agree with the epidemiologic transition theory?' *Demographic Research* 18: 531–68.
Mackenbach, J. P. (1999). 'The Epidemiological Transition Theory'. *Journal of Epidemiology and Community Health* 48: 329–32.
Manderson, L. and Naemiratch, B. (2010). 'From Jollibee to BeeBee: "Lifestyle" and Chronic Illness in Southeast Asia'. *Asia-Pacific Journal of Public Health* 22: 117S-124S.
McKeown, T. (1976). *The modern rise of population*. London: Edward Arnold.
McKeown, T., Brown, R. G. and Record, R. (1972). 'An Interpretation of the Modern Rise of Population in Europe'. *Population Studies-a Journal of Demography* 26: 345–82.
McNeill, W. (1976). *Plagues and Peoples*. Oxford: Blackwell.
Miranda, J. J., Kinra, S. Casas, J., Smith, G. and Ebrahim, S. (2008). 'Non-communicable diseases in low- and middle-income countries: context, determinants and health policy'. *Tropical Medicine and International Health* 13: 1225–34.
Mooney, G. (2007). 'Infectious diseases and epidemiologic transition in Victorian Britain? Definitely'. *Social History of Medicine* 20(3): 595–606.
Nnadozie, E. U. (1995). *Oil and socioeconomic crisis in Nigeria: a regional perspective to the Nigerian disease and the rural sector*. Lewiston, New York: Mellen University Press.
Okonta, I. and Douglas, O. (2003). *Where vultures feast: shell, human rights, and oil in the Niger Delta*. London: Verso.
Olshansky, S. J. and Ault, A. B. (1986). 'The 4th Stage of the Epidemiologic Transition – The Age of Delayed Degenerative Diseases'. *Milbank Quarterly* 64(3): 355–91.

Omran, A. (1971). 'The Epidemiologic Transition: A theory of the epidemiology of population change'. *Milbank Memorial Quarterly* XLIX: 509–38.

Overton, M. (1996) *Agricultural revolution in England: The transformation of the agrarian economy, 1500–1850*. Cambridge; Cambridge University Press.

Ragin, C. C. and Bradshaw, Y. W. (1992). 'International Economic Dependence and Human Misery, 1938–80 – A Global Perspective'. *Sociological Perspectives* 35(2): 217–47.

Rogers, R. G. and Hackenberg, R. (1987). 'Extending epidemiologic transition theory: a new stage'. *Soc Biol* 34(3–4): 234–43.

Salomon, J. A. and Murray, C. J. L. (2002). 'The Epidemiologic Transition Revisited: Compositional Models for Causes of Death by Age and Sex'. *Population and Development Review* 28(2): 205–28.

Savvides, A. and Mohtadi, H. (1991). 'Export Diversification And Export Instability: Some Evidence From South East Asia And Latin America'. *International Economic Journal* 5(1): 15–33.

Shandra, J. M., Nobles, J. London, B. and Williamson, J. (2004). 'Dependency, democracy, and infant mortality: a quantitative, cross-national analysis of less developed countries.' *Social Science 33*.

Shen, C. and Williamson, J. B. (2001). 'Accounting for cross-national differences in infant mortality decline (1965–91) among less developed countries: Effects of women's status, economic dependency, and state strength'. *Social Indicators Research* 53(3): 257–88.

Soutar, G. N. (1977). 'Export Instability and Concentration in Less Developed-Countries – Cross-Sectional Analysis'. *Journal of Development Economics* 4(3): 279–97.

Spijker, J. and Llorens, A. B. (2009). 'Mortality in Catalonia in the context of the third, fourth and future phases of the epidemiological transition theory'. *Demographic Research* 20: 129–67.

Stevens, G., Dias, R. H. et al. (2008). 'Characterizing the Epidemiological Transition in Mexico: National and Subnational Burden of Diseases, Injuries, and Risk Factors'. *PLoS Med* 5(6): e125.

Steverding, D. (2008). 'The history of African trypanosomiasis'. *Parasites & Vectors* 1(1): 3.

Stratton, L., O'Neill, M., Kruk, M. and Bell, M. (2008). 'The persistent problem of malaria: Addressing the fundamental causes of a global killer'. *Social Science & Medicine* 67(5): 854–62.

Stuckler, D. (2008). 'Population causes and consequences of leading chronic diseases: A comparative analysis of prevailing explanations'. *Milbank Quarterly* 86(2): 273–326.

Tegene, A. (1990). 'Commodity Concentration and Export Earnings Instability: The Evidence from African Countries'. *The American Economist* 34: 55–59.

UN-Habitat (2003) *The Challenge of Slums: Global Report on Human Settlements*. London: Earthscan Publications.

Wallerstein, I. M. (1974). *The Modern World-System I: Capitalist Agriculture and the Origins of the European World-Economy in the Sixteenth Century*. New York: Academic Press.

——(1989). *The Modern World-System. Vol III. The Second Era of Great Expansion of the Capitalist World-Economy, 1730s–1840s* New York: Academic Press.

——(2004). *World-systems analysis: an introduction*, Durham, NC: Duke University Press.

Weisz, G. and Olszynko-Gryn, J. (2010). 'The Theory of Epidemiologic Transition: the Origins of a Citation Classic'. *Journal of the History of Medicine and Allied Sciences* 65(3): 287–326.

Wilkinson, R. G. (2001). *Mind the gap: hierarchies, health and human evolution*. London: Yale University Press.

——(2005). *The impact of inequality: how to make sick societies healthier*. Oxford: Routledge.

Wilkinson, R. G. and Pickett, K. (2009). *The spirit level: why more equal societies almost always do better*. London: Allen Lane.

Young, F. W. (1994). 'The Structural Causes of Infant-Mortality Decline in Chile'. *Social Indicators Research* 31(1): 27–46.

8 Archer, morphogenesis and the role of agency in the sociology of health inequalities

Graham Scambler

There is a sense in which agency, or the individual or collective power to *make a difference*, is too readily assumed within sociological discourse on health inequalities. The very choice of health inequalities as a phenomenon appropriate for sociological investigation, together with the presumption that 'appropriate' here implies a purposive commitment to their reduction, are (1) normative, and (2) too frequently pass without comment let alone analysis. Health inequalities, like diseases, are to be eliminated wherever possible, and this is part and parcel of the sociological as well as the public health project. Health inequalities, in short, are in significant measure health *inequities*. In this chapter I argue that a great deal more needs to be said. Drawing on the rigorous and sustained body of work of Margaret Archer, best known as a realist social theorist and sociologist of education, I contend that credible concepts of agency and agential (and transformatory) power are crucial for a sociology of health inequalities; that agency is necessarily structured *but not structurally determined*; and that agency and structure alike need to be analyzed against the backcloth of neo-Marxist notions of 'contradiction'.

Archer's published work can be characterized as critical realist, owing much to the philosopher Roy Bhaskar, but her sociological innovations are uncompromisingly independent (as anyone who knows her would recognize). In this chapter's opening paragraphs I draw on her own exposition of critical realist thought to catch something of its thrust, before venturing into a more detailed account of her sociological appropriation.

Introduction: Archer and critical realism

It seems odd that many researchers of health inequalities need to be reminded that the positivist tradition is seriously flawed and traduces natural and social reality, let alone the differences between them. What realism substitutes for positivism is 'the quest for non-observable generative mechanisms whose powers may exist unexercised or be exercised unrealized, that is with variable outcomes due to the variety of intervening contingencies which cannot be subject to laboratory closure' (Archer, 1998: 190). Society is an open system, and not just in the positivistic sense that it can be difficult to control for extraneous variables (Scambler,

2010). It is open because it is 'necessarily peopled', and its inhabitants are no less reflexive and agential than its investigators.

Gellner (1971) once remarked of social structures that they are, 'I am somewhat sheepishly tempted to say, "really there"'. Bhaskar and Archer are less sheepish. Bhaskar's realism rejects positivism. A social ontology commits itself, if corrigibly, to what exists. In doing so it sets parameters for the explanatory programme. The specification of the constituents (and non-constituents) of what exists 'are the only ones which can appear in explanatory statements (which does not rule out *substantive* debate about the most promising contenders within the abstractly defined domain of the real)' (Archer, 1998: 194). Archer's formula for realism is: 'social ontology (SE) → explanatory methodology (EM) → practical social theories (PST)'.

Archer identifies three ontological premises that are pivotal for realist social theory and comments on their role in the SE → EM → PST formula. The first of these is *intransitivity*. The rejection of positivism rests on substituting an ontology of structures for one of observable events. Moreover, the existence of *intransitive entities*, independent of their identification, is a condition of the possibility of sociology *qua* social science. In the absence of this there could be no explanatory programme. Archer elaborates:

> explanation of social matters requires the generic assertion that there is a state of the matter which is what it is, regardless of how we do view it, choose to view it or are somehow manipulated into viewing it. This precludes any collapse of the ontological into the epistemological and convicts those who endorse this move of the 'epistemic fallacy', namely confusing what is with what we take it to be. Conversely the realist insists that what is the case places limitations upon how we can construe it.
>
> (Archer, 1998: 195)

It does not follow, however, that the social is somehow immutable. On the contrary, a defining feature of society is what Archer terms its 'morphogenetic' nature, that is, its capacity to change its shape or form. What then are the intransitive objects of sociological study? Archer cites Bhaskar (1989: 41) here: 'neither individuals nor groups satisfy the requirement of continuity ... for the autonomy of society over discrete moments of time. In social life only relations endure'. It follows, in other words, that EM realism entails a *relational* conception of the subject matter of social science. Because of its social ontology, realism must give rise to a form of theorizing that transcends the old debate between varieties of methodological individualism and holism.

The second premise is that of *transfactuality*. Mechanisms are continuously active, due to their enduring properties and powers, despite their outcomes displaying variability in open systems. This premise too has entailments. Transfactuality entails that:

> although the form of society at any given time is historically contingent, this is not the same as viewing things social as pure contingency ... only on the

metaphysical assumption that some relations are necessary and at least relatively enduring can we reasonably set out to practise science or to study society ... social realism's acknowledgement that transfactuality is only *relatively* enduring *and* quintessentially *mutable* means that its explanatory programme (EM) has no baggage of preconceptions that society's ordering (at a given time or over time) resembles any other form of reality (mechanism or organism), nor that the totality is homologous with some part of it (language), or some state of it (simple cybernetic systems).

(Archer, 1998: 196)

If it is only contingent that any particular social structure exists, then realist sociology is committed to providing a particular kind of explanation: an analytic history of its emergence.

The final premise is that reality is *stratified*. It is a premise about ontological depth. Three strata require differentiation: the 'surface' stratum of *events*; accessed via the *empirical* stratum of experience; and the stratum of deep, 'beneath-the-surface' or *real* structures. Archer (1998: 196) again:

in terms of the explanatory programme, the stratified nature of reality introduces a necessary historicity (however short the time period involved) for instead of *horizontal* explanations relating one experience, observable or event to another, the fact that these themselves are conditional upon antecedents, requires *vertical* explanation in terms of the generative relationships indispensable for their realisation (and equally necessary to account for the systematic non-actualisation of non-events and non-experiences ...). Ontological depth necessarily introduces vertical causality which simultaneously entails temporality.

The historicity/temporality of vertical explanation is readily illustrated. Religion produces churches not vice versa; and in the absence of 'ideology' imbibed via the practice of shopping, Saatchi and Saatchi could not have presented Thatcher's cuts as 'good housekeeping' (see Collier, 1989). 'When we ask what needs to be the case for x to be possible', 'we predicate any realisation of x upon the *prior* materialisation of the conditions of its possibility' (Archer, 1998: 197). This is what Bhaskar is getting at when he maintains that social forms are a necessary condition for any intentional act, and that their *pre-existence* establishes their *autonomy* as possible objects of scientific investigation.

These premises concerning SO are critical for realist sociology. Archer rightly insists that the effects of a phenomenon like inflation, on spending power for example, are causally influential independently of people's familiarity with economics. 'Pensioners' trade heating against eating regardless of their grasp of index-linked incomes. Crucially for the account of health inequalities that follows, she adds:

I would stress the ways in which structure shapes the situations we confront and also the influential distribution of material and cultural resources with which we can strategically conduct this confrontation. *Some things go on behind*

> *our backs and the effects of many that go on before our faces do not require us to face up to them.*
>
> (Archer, 1998: 199, my emphasis)

Archer cites Porpora's (1989) contention that *positions* must predate the *practices* they engender: the causal effects of structures on individuals are manifested in certain (structured) interests, resources, powers, constraints and predicaments consolidated into each position by the web of relationships. These constitute the 'circumstances' in which people must act and which motivate them to act in certain ways.

Especially relevant to this chapter is Archer's interrogation of *whose* activities, distributions, positions, roles and institutions set the scene for, constrain/enable, others' decision making. Her answer is that they are mostly dead: it is inherited structural and cultural contexts that most effectively condition present actions. Drawing on Bhaskar, she argues that critical realism 'empowers us to analyse the processes by which structure and agency shape and re-shape one another over time and to explain variable outcomes at different times.

(Archer, 1998: 203)

Morphogenesis and more on agency

This chapter takes off from Archer's morphogenetic approach and is in a sense an elaboration of it; but its targets are specific. A brief summation of morphogenesis will therefore suffice. Allied to the case for vertical over horizontal explanation is a need to analytically decouple structure and agency, 'so as to examine their *mutual interplay across time*; something which can result both in *stable reproduction* or *change* through the emergence of new properties and powers' (Williams, 1999: 809). Only on the basis of such a decoupling, Archer insists, does it become possible to explore the interface between structure and agency on which social theory depends. Structure and agency, Bhaskar (1989: 92) argues, are:

> ... existentially interdependent but essentially distinct. Society is both ever-present *condition* and continually reproduced *outcome* of human agency: this is the duality of structure. And human agency is both work (generically conceived), that is, (normatively conscious) *production*, and (normatively unconscious) *reproduction* of the conditions of production, including society: this is the duality of praxis.

Bhaskar's articulation of what he calls the 'transformational model of social action' underpins Archer's (1995) morphogenetic model. In her terms, *structural conditioning* necessarily pre-dates actions that either reproduce (that is, are *morphostatic*) or elaborate on structures (that is, are *morphogenetic*), and concerning which humans may or may not be reflexive in the course of *socio-cultural interaction*.

Arguing against 'postmodern' explications of the body and of disease, Williams (1999: 806) draws on Bhaskar and Archer to make another point relating to structure and agency of particular salience to this chapter. He insists that the body, 'diseased or otherwise', is a real entity ('no matter what we call it or how we observe it'). The objection here is to the 'epistemic fallacy', or the reduction of (a) what exists to (b) what we do or can know of what exists. The body, Williams maintains, 'has its own mind-independent generative structures and causal mechanisms. As such it has an ontological depth independent of epistemological claims, right or wrong, as to its existence'.

Our embodied nature as a 'species-being' not only constrains who can become a person, it has direct implications too for what a person can do. Archer (1995: 288) again:

> ... the characteristics of homo sapiens (as a natural kind) cannot be attributed to society, even if they can only be exercised within in. On the contrary, human beings must have a particular physical constitution for them to be consistently socially influenced (as in learning speech, arithmetic, tool making). Even in cases where the biological may be socially mediated in almost every instance or respect ... this does not mean that the mediated is not biological nor that the physical becomes epiphenomenal.

Humans, I have argued in a similar vein, are simultaneously the products of biological, psychological and social mechanisms, whilst yet retaining their agency; on top of this are the sometimes mundane and sometimes dramatic interruptions of contingency (e.g. on the latter end of the spectrum, the volcanic destruction of Pompeii and most of its citizenry and the recent devastation in Japan occasioned by an earthquake and tsunami). Humans can be said to be biologically, psychologically and social 'structured' *without being structurally determined* (Scambler et al., 2010). So what is left for agency and its transformative power?

Reflexivity in action

> The subjective powers of reflexivity mediate the role that objective structural or cultural powers play in influencing social action and are thus indispensable to explaining social outcomes.
>
> (Archer, 2007: 5)

Agency is necessarily contextualized. Archer's (1995, 2003, 2007) way of articulating this is in terms of a three-stage model (see Figure 8.1). It is in light of such a model that individual reflexivity must be broached. Vygotsky (1934) argued that while external speech is for others, 'inner speech' is for oneself. In her *Structure, Agency and the Internal Conversation* (2003) Archer constructs a detailed defence of this notion of an 'internal conversation'. She argues that:

(1) it is a genuinely *interior* phenomenon, and one that underwrites the private life of the social subject;
(2) its subjectivity has a first-person ontology, precluding any attempt to render it in the third-person; and
(3) it possesses *causal efficacy*.

In her *Making our Way through the World* (Archer 2007: 64) she builds on her defence of this 'inner reflexive dialogue' to focus on its exercise as a power by ordinary people negotiating their lives. Her 'guiding hypothesis' is that 'the interplay between people's nascent "concerns" (the importance of what they care about) and their "context" (the continuity or discontinuity of their social environment) shapes the mode of reflexivity they regularly practice' (Archer, 2007: 96). It is the application of her philosophical and theoretical ideas that is of interest here. The next few paragraphs are given over to a consideration of her elaboration and deployment of the idea of an internal conversation, after which its potential to illuminate our understanding of the salience of agency in health inequalities research is discussed.

Archer accepts Wiley's (2004) judgement that the methodological obstacles to accessing inner reflexive dialogue are not insurmountable: 'semantic privacy does not prevent one from describing one's own inner speech to another, at least to a substantial extent'. On this basis, and with diligence and caution, Archer discerns in participants in her studies four modes of reflexivity. This affords the following ideal types: *communicative reflexives, autonomous reflexives, meta-reflexives* and *fractured reflexives*. These are defined in Table 8.1.

She reserves further analysis of fractured reflexives for a future volume, but this need not constrain us here. Her ideal typical elaboration of communicative, autonomous and meta-reflexives can be paraphrased as follows:

- *Communicative reflexives* remain embedded in the ('natal') circumstances of their entry into the social world. They 'evade' both the objective costs that would be incurred in resisting constraints and the bonuses associated with enablements, the combined effect of which is to leave them immobile.
- *Autonomous reflexives* adopt a strategic approach towards constraints and enablements, seeking to avoid 'snakes' and climb 'ladders'. Their aspiration is to improve their position, and if successful they are upwardly mobile.
- *Meta-reflexives* are subversive in relation to constraints and enablements 'because of their willingness to pay the price of the former and to forfeit the benefits of the latter in the attempt to live out their ideal' (Archer, 2007: 98). Social volatility is the predictable result.

The micro-political life politics of individuals contribute to the 'macroscopic' structuring and restructuring of society. In general, the combined day-to-day practices of communicative reflexives comprise the cement of society. The autonomous reflexives, for their part, combine to foster social development by injecting dynamism into the new positions they occupy. They are the source of productivity in its multifarious aspects. Collectively, the meta-reflexives 'function as the well-spring of society's social criticism': they underwrite Weber's realm of *Wertrationalitat*, or value rationality (Archer, 2007: 99).

Ideal types not only admit but entail exception and complexity. Ideal typical assignment is the start not the end of the story for each individual. More needs to be said here of each of Archer's ideal types.

1   Structural and cultural properties *objectively* shape the situations that agents confront involuntarily, and *inter alia* possess generative powers of constraint and enablement in relation to
2   The subject's own constellations of concerns, as *subjectively* defined in relation to the three orders of natural reality: nature, practice and the social.
3   Courses of action are produced through the *reflexive deliberations* of subjects who *subjectively* determine their practical projects in relation to their *objective* circumstances.

Figure 8.1 The three-stage model

(A) Communicative reflexives

We all engage in communicative reflexivity, but only for some is it the dominant mode of reflexivity. What is distinctive about the internal conversation of communicative reflexives is that its conclusion requires the input of others: intra-subjectivity needs to be supplemented by inter-subjectivity (Archer, 2007: 102). Given our natal or initially 'involuntary' placement in society, these 'others' are typically recruited from those who comprise communicative reflexives' local peers or reference group, hence the tendency to social immobility.

(B) Autonomous reflexives

The internal conversations of autonomous reflexives, by contrast, are self-contained affairs. The lone inner dialogue is sufficient here to determine a course of action. When this is the dominant mode of reflexivity, those involved neither seek nor require the involvement of others in their decision making. Of course autonomous reflexives also engage in communicative reflexivity, but this is for them not strictly necessary. 'Whilst the autonomous subject may respond readily, articulately

Table 8.1 Modes of reflexivity

Modes	Description
Communicative reflexives	Those whose internal conversations require completion and confirmation by others before resulting in courses of action.
Autonomous reflexives	Those who sustain self-contained internal conversations, leading directly to action.
Meta-reflexives	Those who are critically reflexive about their own internal conversations and critical about effective action in society.
Fractured reflexives	Those whose internal conversations intensify their distress and disorientation rather than leading to purposeful courses of action.

Source: Archer (2007)

and take interest in the reactions of others, none of these interchanges is driven by need' (Archer, 2007: 114).

(C) Meta-reflexives

The notion of meta-reflexivity, implying reflection on reflection, may seem abstruse, even narcissistic, but self-monitoring is part and parcel of day-to-day living. In those for whom it is the dominant mode meta-reflexivity is a routine kind of self-questioning. 'Why did I say that?' 'Why am I so reticent to say what I think?' Meta-reflexives are 'conversant with their own reflexivity'. They are self-critical and tend to be preoccupied with the moral worth of their projects and their worthiness to undertake them.

Nothing has been said yet of Archer's fourth ideal type, the *fractured reflexives*, save for the definition in Table 8.1; this, it will be remembered, is because she plans to accord them a volume of their own. Two of their characteristics are relevant here however. First, fractured reflexivity lends itself to passive agency, unlike the triad that Archer focuses on in *Making our Way through the World*. For fractured reflexives, internal conversation typically leads to disorientation and distress: their deliberations go round in circles and lack conclusions. And second, it is communicative reflexives who are most fragile and vulnerable to displacement into the category of fractured reflexive (the majority or fractured reflexives in Archer's study sample started out as communicative reflexives).

Building on Archer's analysis, and with a passing nod to Habermas (1984, 1987), it is suggested here that communicative reflexives are (communicatively) oriented to 'consensus'; autonomous reflexives are (strategically) orientated to 'outcome'; meta-reflexives are oriented to 'values'; and fractured reflexives are non- or disoriented.

Sociology, health inequalities and the GBH

Arguably the sociology of health inequalities has of late been less challenging and assertive than the socio-epidemiology of health inequalities. It has certainly been less ambitious (Scambler, 2012). It will be taken as read in this chapter that a 'statistical' association between assorted socio-economic classifications (SECs) and health and longevity has been established beyond dispute (see WHO, 2008; The Marmot Report, 2010): essentially, the lower one's SEC the poorer one's fortunes. Behavioural, material and psychosocial variables, and mechanisms, as well as specific junctures of the life course (notably childhood), have been postulated as causally critical. I have maintained elsewhere that, in contradistinction to much ongoing study, the optimum *sociological* route to understanding and explaining health inequalities is not via endlessly replicated empirical investigations of the poor and powerless, but rather through a more nuanced understanding and explanation of the day-to-day decision making of the rich and powerful. The 'greedy bastards hypothesis' (GBH) points the causal finger at a strongly globalized 'cabal' at the apex of a capitalist executive comprising the strategic decision makers in the economy. This cabal holds sway over the state's as yet more weakly globalized power elite; and thereby indirectly and circuitously saps the health, health-related quality of life and life expectancy of those who serve it (Scambler, 2007, 2009, 2012).

If there is any substance to the polemically framed GBH, then Archer's critical realist sociology of the causal efficacy of agency in general, and of reflexivity and the internal conversation in particular, has considerable potential. It sits somewhere between the philosophical assertion of free will and what Archer takes to be Bourdieu's sociological but overly socialized or structured notion of *habitus*. The GBs of the GBH, I shall suggest, are a distinctive and socio-/psychopathological subset of Archer's autonomous reflexives.

The GBH is part and parcel of the post-1970s class/command dynamic. An analysis developed elsewhere (Scambler, 2001; Scambler, 2002, 2007, 2009) is summarized in Figure 8.2. For present purposes more needs to be said about the parameters and memberships of the 'British' capitalist-executive cabal (CEC) and power elite (PE), representing class and command relations respectively.

(A) Capitalist-executive cabal

According to the neo-Gramscian perspective of the 'Amsterdam Project' (van der Pijl, 1984), capitalism's trajectory has been characterized by a series of 'concepts of control', each of which offers a paradigm for managing capitalism from a particular fractional standpoint. The functional division of capital into industrial and financial forms gives rise to the *productive capital concept* and the *money capital concept* respectively. Carroll (2008) notes a growing tension between industrial and financial capital: there is a contradiction between capital as surplus value production (epitomized by the management of industry) and capital as abstract labour (epitomized by mobile money capital). If postwar organized or Fordist capitalism saw banking and rentier interests subordinated to productive capital – via financial regulations, capital controls and so on – the 'crisis' of Fordism in the early 1970s, together with the rise of neo-liberal policies, 'set in motion a restructuring that would recompose the bourgeoisie's dominant stratum' (Carroll, 2008: 53).

In the 1970s the US abrogation of Bretton Woods and the rise of the Eurodollar freed money capital from national regulation by central banks, and international recession drew banks further into the global arena. This led to the emergence of transnational finance as international banks established closer relations with transnational corporations; and also to the resurgence of money capital – and of the money capital concept of control – in the leading capitalist economies (Carroll, 2008). Commentators wrote about processes of *financialization*, alluding not only to deregulation and internationalization, but also to a shift in the distribution of profits from productive money to money capital, accompanied by an increase in the external financing of industry, and to a reorientation, deeply penetrating 'industrial' corporations, towards the financial sphere. Carroll (2008: 55–56) again: ' ... the constellation of interests atop major firms has shifted from salaried managers and bankers, towards institutional shareholders and, at certain junctures of corporate restructuring, private equity outfits'. Industrial capital, in short, has increasingly come to resemble financial capital 'as stock options align corporate management with a money-capital standpoint and as firms ... come to depend less on productive activities and more on income from financial sources'. In the financial sector meanwhile, deregulation has precipitated capital centralization in banks with global reach 'whose activities range from financial production to speculation in derivatives', while 'institutional investors controlling capitalized deferred wages (have) become important centres of allocative as well as strategic power' (Carroll, 2008: 56). And then came the global financial crisis of 2008/2009.

So the 'British' CEC has a different character from its predecessors in Fordist and pre-Fordist times. Needless to say, its membership is not picked up in population-wide, employment-based operationalizations of class or putative proxies like SECs; rather, it goes missing and remains under-investigated, not least in relation to the GBH. What needs to be emphasized is not only the financialization of post-Fordist capitalism, but also the growing interpenetration of previously nation-bound capital executives, warranting the assertion of a transnational CEC in the making (Sklair, 2000). There is no need to postulate an international or inter-cabalistic conspiracy since there has as yet been so little necessity to conspire under the global neo-liberal orthodoxy of financial capitalism.

(B) State power elite

In financial capitalism members of Britain's CEC have come to exercise a growing sway over what Oborne (2007) presciently calls its (individualized, career-oriented and philosophically flexible) 'political class', which is located at the core of the complex, regulatory and 'colonizing' apparatus of the state. The PE is neither easier to define definitively nor to operationalize than the CEC. It comprises more than the prime minister and his coterie of advisers, the cabinet, ministers of state or even Oborne's political class as a whole. The *vertical* or 'Westminster' model of the PE has been displaced by a model resting on theories of the *horizontal* distribution of power and overlapping networks (Rhodes, 1995). Smith (1999: 33–35) interprets command relations in terms of 'resource dependency':

> Frequently, outcomes can be a positive-sum game rather than a zero-sum one. In order to achieve goals, actors have to negotiate, compromise and bargain. Consequently, power does not just exist in conflicts between cabinet and Prime Minister but, as Foucault suggests, it is in every situation and relationship as actors develop belief systems, strategies and alliances in order to exchange resources and achieve goals. There is no need to adopt a discourse or post-modern approach to see the core executive as a field of micro-politics, where power is exercised through a multitude of agencies and coherence imposed through the 'adoption of shared vocabularies'.

Shrewd Foucauldian insights into 'how' power is exercised should not tempt us, however, to abandon 'why' questions, the focus of the class/command dynamic emphasized in this contribution. Micro-politics do not occur in a structural vacuum. What Smith (2009) has recently described as the *past*modern state has

(A) Theses
- In the terminology of French regulation theory, regimes of capital accumulation (involving relations of class), and their concomitant modes of regulation (involving relations of command), tend to increases in inequalities of wealth and income, even when flows of material assets are strengthening across the population as a whole.
- The regime of capital accumulation/mode of regulation prevailing since the 1970s has seen a particularly steep increase in material inequality occasioned in significant part by the newly asymmetrical dynamic of class-based exploitation and state or command-based oppression.
- These two theses are fundamental to a credible sociology of health inequalities (and paradoxically help explain why we currently lack one in Britain).
- The endlessly replicated statistical linkages between SECs and other proxies for class and health and longevity, coalescing in the notion of the 'social gradient', bear transfactual, retroductive testimony both to the existence of relations of class and to their causal efficacy for health.
- Neo-liberalism's state-sanctioned policy of 'personal responsibility' (presented via concepts like 'behavioural conditionality') affords ideological cover for the post-1970s regime of capital accumulation/mode of regulation.
- The GBH highlights the structural, causal–explanatory contribution of the present class/command dynamic to: (a) the increasingly unequal division of material asset flows; and, in part a result of (a), (b) the reduction in other asset flows pivotal for health and longevity *that cluster in low-income households* (see below).

(B) 'Asset flows' of causal salience for health status and longevity
- *Material assets* refer in developed societies to 'relative deprivation' due to impoverishment and meagre standards of living. The relevance of material assets has long been stressed, although the mechanisms linking low income with health remain much debated.
- *Biological (or body) assets* can be affected by class even prior to birth: low-income families are more likely to produce low-birth-weight babies; and low-birth-weight babies carry an increased risk of chronic disease in childhood, possibly through biological programming.
- *Psychological assets* yield a generalized capacity to cope, extending to what is increasingly conceptualized as resilience. The 'vulnerability factors' found to reduce women's capacity to cope with those life events salient for depression can be seen as class-induced interruptions to the flow of psychological assets (Brown and Harris, 1978).
- *Social assets*, often termed 'social capital', refer to aspects of social integration, networks and support.
- *Cultural assets*, constituting 'cultural capital', are generated initially through processes of primary socialization and go on to embrace educational opportunity and attainment. Arrests to a class-related cultural asset flow can have long-term detrimental effects on employment and income levels, and therefore on health.
- *Spatial assets* have been shown to be significant for health via area-based studies revealing that areas of high mortality tend to be areas with high rates of net out-migration; and it is the better qualified and more affluent who exercise the option to move.
- *Symbolic assets* refer to the variable distribution of status or honour and are known to impact on people's health, notably via their sense of social position and accomplishment relative to their reference groups (Marmot, 2006).

Figure 8.2 The theory so far

142 *Graham Scambler*

modern foundations. States cannot altogether escape the Hobbesian problem of order, as was apparent during the 2008–09 banking crisis. I have argued that they have under the tutelage of the CEC become *more* regulatory whilst deploying novel mechanisms (Scambler, 2007). Smith (2009: 266) writes:

> What we have seen in recent years has been the development of new and powerful mechanisms of control by states. These mechanisms have focussed on surveillance, risk, rationality and regulation.

For all that the British PE retains functions of its own (that is, is not simply an epiphenomenon of class), it has become far more compliant with its CEC. In fact, as current, cross-political party machinations to 'reform' the English and Welsh National Health Service (NHS) reveal, the clandestine cooperation between PE and CEC stretching back to the early 1990s is a symptom of personal interests readily allied to class interests (witness the machinations of New Labour's Patricia Hewitt and Alan Milburn) (Leys and Player, 2011).

In the next section I characterize the British CEC and PE in terms of Archer's notion of the internal conversation. This leads to an *a priori* (rather than empirical, *pace* Archer) identification of a possible sub-type of autonomous reflexive. In the chapter's concluding paragraphs the potential of this provisional analysis for contributing to a more comprehensive sociology of health inequalities is considered.

CEC, PE and autonomous reflexivity

The GBs constituting the CEC exert their influence through the PE and are buttressed by 'strategists' in the capitalist executive as a whole, as well as by 'tacticians' recruited from the new (and to a lesser extent old) middle classes. That they are 'greedy bastards' may need a word of elaboration since this concept is not part of a familiar sociological lexicon. There is no doubting the voracity of their appetites. According to the Interim Report of the High Pay Commission (High Pay Commission, 2011), those who make up the lion's share of 'Britain's' top 0.1 per cent earners are finance and business workers and company directors. FTSE 100 chief executives enjoyed average total remuneration of over £4.2 million in 2009/2010. In 2010, FTSE 100 CEO pay was 145 times the average salary for workers, and it is on track to be 214 times the average salary for workers by 2020. Given this frequently unearned and serendipitous boost for the 'super-rich', ranging from *gambling* financiers to CEOs and directors rewarded for downsizing, outsourcing, privatizing, closing or undermining workers' pension schemes, and so on (Scambler, 2009), it would be churlish to deny greed. So much for the adjective. The noun acknowledges that the super-rich are beneficiaries of one of capitalism's core contradictions: it is the enhanced exploitation of the labour of others that feeds as well as helps satisfy their apparently insatiable appetites (see Scambler and Scambler, forthcoming).

Three points might be appended to this definitional statement before the CEC, and in a slightly different sense, the PE are associated with a specific sub-type of autonomous reflexivity. The first draws on a distinction made elsewhere between stigma, denoting an infringement of norms of *shame*, and deviance, marking an infringement of norms of *blame* (Scambler, 2009). The only reason 'benefit cheats' are widely chastised by the CEC, PE and their allies, that is, shamed and/or blamed, *and the globally nomadic tax-avoiding/tax-evading GBs are not*, is because the latter have the money and power to make their charges plausible and 'stickable' while the former do not (Link and Phelan, 2001). As the bankers demonstrated in 2008/2009, the GBs can do almost anything without being *effectively* shamed and/ or blamed (Scambler, 2009). By way of an aside, by what criteria is it acceptable for the Duke of Westminster to inherit the means to forgo labour entirely while others born less privileged *must*, on pain of financial retribution, respond positively to a CEC/PE-sponsored and policed 'imperative to work'? Justifications or 'excusing conditions' are rarely required of GBs in a post-Fordist, post-welfare statist *and postmodern or relativized culture* that allows neo-liberal ideology to prevail as a ubiquitous but seemingly non-opposable or default 'petit narrative' (Scambler, 2002). A postmodern or relativized culture, as Habermas (1987b) observes, is intrinsically conservative. In Southwood's (2011) eloquent phrase, it is a culture of 'non-stop inertia'.

The second point is that the GBH represents a sociological not a personal stance (Scambler, 2009). In other words, those who make up the CEC/PE are replaceable rather than, as neo-liberal ideology would have it, exceptionally charismatic, shrewd and daring and therefore 'irreplaceable'. Their sociological significance, not least for health inequalities, is that they are 'surfers' of social structures and relations of class and command.

The third point draws on the work of Habermas (1984, 1987a) to posit a learned predisposition to strategic as opposed to communicative action on the part of the GBs. Habermas argues that in modern, highly differentiated societies 'system' (economy and state) and 'lifeworld' (private/household and public/deliberative spheres) have become 'de-coupled'; and the former, via their 'steering media' of money and power, have increasingly come to dominate or 'colonize' the latter (see Edwards, this volume). In the less complex era of *The Prince*, Machiavelli discerned an incompatibility between the goals and practices of the statesman and the (Christian) moralist. In contemporary and Habermasian terms, the former was essentially strategic, the latter essentially communicative. Members of the CEC, and increasingly of the PE, are likewise 'essentially strategic'. Their orientations to outcome via fixations on money and power respectively squeeze out or render residual any commitment to consensus: morality becomes a largely strategic issue, subordinated to short-term financial, business or political agendas.

It was suggested earlier that the CEC and PE include a disproportionate share of distinctive autonomous reflexives. I shall use the term '*focused* autonomous reflexives' to capture this special sub-type. Before spelling out the core elements of this Weberian ideal type it bears repeating that the GBs of the CEC and PE are of course not exclusive in their greed or instrumental use of others, far from it (Scambler, 2009). No more do they exhaust the sub-type of focused autonomous reflexives outlined here. But the structuring of their internal conversations is certainly pertinent to a sociology of health inequalities that accords due weight, belatedly, to wealth and power, as well as to the simultaneous exercise of structure and agency.

The six core constituents of the focused autonomous reflexive, for present purposes illustrated in terms of the CEC and PE, are:

- *Total commitment*

The focused autonomous reflexive exhibits an overriding engagement with accumulating capital (and personal wealth/income) (CEC) or power (PE). Nothing less will suffice: that is, any deficit in commitment will result in absolute or relative failure.

- *Nietzschean instinct*

Born of a Hobbesian notion of the natural human state, the commitment of the CEC/PE betrays a ruthless determination to cut whatever corners are necessary to gain advantage over rivals.

- *Fundamentalist ideology*

The commitment of the CEC/PE is not only total and Nietzschean but fundamentalist: it does not admit of compromise. It is an ideology – that is, a standpoint emerging from a coherent set of vested (class/command) interests – that brooks no alternative.

- *Cognitive insurance*

While cognitive dissonance is a state to which none of us is immune, the CEC/PE is able, courtesy of the new class/command dynamic, to take out sufficient insurance to draw its sting. Thus accusations of greed and responsibility for others' suffering are rarely internalized. Such epistemological and ontological security is the exception rather than the rule in this era.

- *Tunnel vision*

A concomitant of a total, Nietzschean and fundamentalist commitment is the sidelining of other matters and a reflex and often gendered delegation of these to others.

- *Lifeworld detachment*

The colonizer is colonized: there is simply no time for the ordinary business of day-to-day decision making. In this way members of the CEC/PE rely on and reproduce structures not only of gender but of class, ethnicity, ageing and so on. Lifeworld detachment presupposes other's non-detachment.

These six characteristics, it is suggested, make up a plausible and sociologically useful ideal type of the focused autonomous reflexive. In the context of this chapter and explication, those who comprise the CEC and PE are a ready fit. It remains now to consider the salience of this analysis for the sociology of health inequalities.

Comments on the sociology of health inequalities

These concluding paragraphs are organized around the notions of 'ideology' on the one hand and 'resistance' on the other. The theme that runs through them is that of the potentially transformative power of (structured but not structurally determined) agency.

(A) Ideology

That people have beliefs, values and attitudes that owe more to their natal or involuntary placement in society than to the exercise of agency seems as much an anachronism in sociology now as it was once a platitude. As much is central to Bhaskar's and Archer's realism, although, crucially, both allow for the exceptional, transformational power of agency. We shall return to the idea of the 'exceptional' when discussing resistance. As far as the CEC/PE dyad is concerned, it should not be surprising that they are the prime peddlers, via mass media and think tanks, of a neo-liberal ideology that either applauds or excuses the GBs of the GBH. Echoing Engels' and Virschow's revolutionary opposition to the bourgeois ideologies of their times and places, to undermine the health and longevity of the poor and powerless by cutting off vital asset flows is no lesser a crime than murder, or at least manslaughter (Scambler, 2012). The role of 'symbolic', indirect or circuitous as opposed to overt physical violence in producing and reproducing health inequalities has been much neglected. Accusations of deviance on the part of the CEC/PE have intermittently been levelled, notably after the financial crash of 2008/2009, but the means have yet to become available to accusers to make the charges stick.

The ideology of *sociological* significance, in other words, is the ideology of the capitalists, the bourgeoisie, the 'neo-cons', the CEC/PE and so on. It is one thing to inherit interests that run 'with' the structural/ideological flow, another to inherit interests that run 'against' them. This was a commonplace of classical sociology. To reintroduce the concept of ideology is necessarily to reintroduce that of 'false consciousness' (Runciman, 1970). Any sociological 'discomfort' at doing so is itself a function of the (ideological) 'taming' of the discipline (Scambler, 1996).

(B) Resistance

Resistance necessarily involves countering, subverting and ultimately undermining the global/national/local potency of ideology, in the present era the ideology of neo-liberalism. And the accumulated evidence of the post-welfare statist decades (mid 1970s onwards) leads ineluctably to the conclusion that health inequalities in the UK (and elsewhere) cannot be addressed effectively by piecemeal social engineering: meaningful resistance in relation to health inequalities *necessarily* reaches deep down into generative social mechanisms, be they of structure *or agency*. The class/command dynamic that characterizes the present represents the key and overriding structural input into health inequalities/inequities. But what of the transformative power of agency?

For Archer (2007: 155), meta-reflexives (oriented by values) are characterized by 'contextual incongruity': this denotes an incongruity between dreams and aspirations and contextual factors that obstruct their realization. But not all dreams fade and die, and those organizers and leaders of resistance to neo-liberal ideology might be said to represent a sub-set of meta-reflexives whose value-driven commitments become central to identity for self and others and transmute into life-long advocacy on behalf of the 'community as a whole'. I shall call them *dedicated meta-reflexives*.

It might superficially appear that these activists resemble the CEC/PE contingent of focused autonomous reflexives; but they are poles apart. While the focused autonomous reflexives are almost entirely instrumental, strategically and ruthlessly oriented to the pursuit of their own interests, the dedicated meta-reflexives are value, other and community or 'third sector' oriented (Archer, 2007: 312). As Archer (2007: 262) shows, the:

> ... meta-reflexive concern for 'community', despite its varied meanings, is light years removed from both the communicative reflexives' preoccupation with their own micro-life worlds and the autonomous reflexives' use of the locality as a place for out-sourcing and paid access to selected facilities ... what unites (meta-reflexives) is not a burgeoning communitarianism, but rather a common belief that social problems will not yield to individualistic incentives or to centralized political interventions.

So where do these paragraphs on ideology and resistance leave us, how do they feed into a more promising sociology of health inequalities? The literature on health inequalities reveals a 'widening gap' with respect to measures of SEC and health and longevity during the unfolding of 'high', 'late' or 'second' modernity since the mid 1970s. While it is neither necessary nor morally appropriate to abandon sociological and other evidence-based inputs into policy formation and implementation, it needs to be recognized that this is often to swim ineffectually against a strengthening tide: when push comes to shove, evidence-based policy metamorphoses into policy-based evidence. This is acknowledged in recent discussions arising out of The Marmot Report (2010). 'No reviews or policies', Pickett and Dorling (2010: 1233) rightly proclaim, '"boldly go" where all public health researchers know they need to go'.

So when Marmot cites Neruda's injunction to 'rise up with me against the organization of misery', a global rather than national or local call to arms, is this a call for revolutionary change? To revisit the opening paragraph of this chapter, what is the degree of commitment to *making a difference*? Eagleton (2011: 19) summarizes:

> Reform is vital; but sooner or later you will hit a point where the system refuses to give way, and for Marxism this is known as the social relations of production. Or, in less polite technical language, a dominant class which control the material resources and is markedly reluctant to hand them over. It is only then that a decisive choice between reform and revolution looms up.

If Marmot and sociologists of health inequalities are serious, then there will have to be a sociological reckoning with the contradictions of capitalism and the likes of transnational and national relations of class and command, a step well beyond an esoteric fascination with SECs. The SEC/health association cannot be explained sociologically in the absence of a comprehensive theory of social class and 'class struggle' (Coburn, 2009; Scambler, 2012; Scambler and Scambler, forthcoming).

Concluding remarks

This chapter draws on one aspect of the recent writings of Margaret Archer, her empirically anchored analysis of reflexivity and humans' 'internal conversations'. This represents a deepening of her previous, critical realist 'morphogenetic theory'. I have maintained elsewhere that a sociology of health inequalities risks being tamed almost beyond redemption in the absence of a macro-theory of social structure, emphasizing the growing salience since the mid 1970s of the class/command dynamic. Peoples' behaviours are structured without being *structurally determined*. (They are similarly and simultaneously structured by biological and psychological as well as social relations, of course, but it is beyond the scope of this chapter to elaborate on this – see Scambler *et al.*, 2010). I have here tried to suggest how agency too is structured without being structurally determined. I can see no conceivable circumstances in which agency is entirely lost to, as opposed to being cruelly constrained by, structures (indeed, to recall Wittgenstein, it could not – logically – survive such a possibility: the one implies the other). So there exists a residual transformatory potential in the agency of all, and much more in the agency of a few.

What Archer's typology of autonomous, communicative, meta- and fractured reflexives permits is a credible *sociology* of agency for a sociology of health inequalities. Consistently with the GBH, I have spent most time on the CEC/PE, leading to the construction of a sub-type of autonomous reflexives, namely, the *focused autonomous reflexives*. The GBs belong in without exhausting this sub-type. The kernel of the argument has been that the tiny minority of 'greedy bastards' who decisively shape the economy, and indirectly the state, exercise structured not unstructured agency: their socio-/psychopathology has social (and possibly also biological and psychological) roots. But in Habermasian terminology, their strategic orientation overcomes and ultimately subdues their communicative orientation to those with whom they interact as well as *deal*.

A by-product of this analysis has been a suggestion that those most likely to promote the kind of revolutionary shift Marmot aspires to comprise part of a sub-type of *dedicated meta-reflexives*. While for want of space no ideal type of the dedicated meta-reflexive has been constructed, it remains a promising concept for empirical enquiry. Another avenue for research might involve Archer's fractured reflexives, many of them former communicative reflexives, who are perhaps both most vulnerable to health problems and a key focus of potential resistance. The general message of this chapter, however, is that the differential structuring of agency is an important but neglected component of any comprehensive sociology of health inequalities, and that Archer's analysis offers an interesting and viable frame for elaboration. The field of morphogenetic action has been largely abandoned by sociologists of health inequalities, many of whom appear to have signed up to an ideological device of policy-based evidence and to be in denial over its usurpation by a praxis of policy-based evidence. The causal efficacy of our internal conversations is a lead worth following.

References

Archer, M. (1995) *Realist Social Theory: The Morphogenetic Approach*. Cambridge: Cambridge University Press.
——(1998) Realism in the social sciences. In Archer, M., Bhaskar, R., Collier, A., Lawson, T. and Norrie, A. (eds) *Critical realism: Basic Readings*. London: Routledge.
——(2003) *Structure, Agency and the Internal Conversation*. Cambridge: Cambridge University Press.
——(2007) *Making our Way through the World*. Cambridge: Cambridge University Press.
Bhaskar, R. (1989a) *The Possibility of Naturalism*. Hemel Hempstead: Harvester.
——(1989b) *Reclaiming Reality*. London: Verso.
Brown, G. and Harris, T. (1978) *Social Origins of Depression*. London: Tavistock.
Carroll, W. (2008) The corporate elite and the transformation of financial capital: a view from Canada. In Savage, M. and Williams, K. (eds) *Remembering Elites*. Oxford: Blackwell.
Coburn, D. (2009) Inequality and health. In Panitch, L. and Leys, C. (eds) *Morbid Symptoms: Health under Capitalism. Socialist Register 2010*. Pontypool: Merlin Press.
Collier, A. (1989) *Scientific Realism and Socialist Thought*. Hemel Hempstead: Harvester Wheatsheaf.
Eagleton, T. (2011) *Why Marx was Right*. New Haven, CT: Yale University Press.
Gellner, E. (1971) Holism versus individualism. In Brodbeck, M. (ed.) *Readings in the Philosophy of the Social Sciences*. New York: Macmillan.
Habermas, J. (1984) *Theory of Communicative Action. Vol. 1: Reason and Rationalization of Society*. London: Heinemann.
——(1987a) *Theory of Communicative Action. Vol. 2: Lifeworld and System: A Critique of Functionalist Reason*. Cambridge: Polity Press.
——(1987b) *The Philosophical Discourse of Modernity*. Cambridge: Polity Press.
High Pay Commission (2011) *More for Less: What has Happened to Pay at the Top and Does it Matter?* London: High Pay Commission.
Leys, C. and Player, S. (2011) *The Plot against the NHS*. Pontypool: Merlin Press.
Link, B. and Phelan, J. (2001) Conceptualizing stigma. *Annual Review of Sociology* 27: 363–85.
Marmot, M. (2006) *Status Syndrome*. London: Bloomsbury.

Oborne, P. (2007) *The Triumph of the Political Class*. London: Simon & Schuster.
Pickett, K. and Dorling, D. (2010) Against the Organization of Misery The Marmot Review of health inequalities. *Social Science and Medicine* 71: 1231–33.
Porpora, D. (1989) Four concepts of social structure. *Journal for the Theory of Social Behaviour* 19: 206.
Rhodes, R. (1995) From Prime Ministerial power to core executive. In Rhodes, R. and Dunleavy, P. (eds) *Prime Minister, Cabinet and Core Executive*. London; Macmillan.
Runciman, W. (1970) *Sociology in its Place and Other Essays*. Cambridge: Cambridge University Press.
Scambler; G. (1996) The 'project modernity' and the parameters for a critical sociology: an argument with illustrations from medical sociology. *Sociology* 30: 567–81.
——(2001) Class, power and the durability of health inequalities. In Scambler, G. (ed.) *Habermas, Critical Theory and Health*. London: Routledge.
——(2002) *Health and Social Change: a Critical Theory*. Buckingham: Open University Press.
——(2007) Social structure and the production, reproduction and durability of health inequalities. *Social Theory and Health* 5: 297–315.
——(2009) Capitalism, workers, profit-making and the sociology of health inequalities. *Social Theory and Health* 7: 17–128.
——(2010) Qualitative and quantitative methodologies in comparative research: an integrated approach? *Salute e Societa* Anno IX Supplemento al n.: 21–37.
——(2012) Review article: health inequalities. *Sociology of Health and Illness*. 34: 130–46.
Scambler, G. and Scambler, S. (forthcoming) Marx and health inequalities. In Cockerham, W. (ed.) *Medical Sociology on the Move*. New York: Springer Press
Scambler, G., Afentouli, P. and Selai, C. (2010) Living with epilepsy: catching simultaneity in the biological, the psychological and the social. In Scambler, G. and Scambler, S. (eds) *New Directions in the Sociology of Chronic and Disabling Conditions: Assaults on the Lifeworld*. London: Palgrave.
Sklair, L. (2000) *The Transnational Capitalist Class*. Cambridge: Polity Press.
Smith, M. (1999) *The Core Executive in Britain*. London: Macmillan.
——(2009) *Power and the State*. London: Palgrave Macmillan.
Southwood, I. (2011) *Non-Stop Inertia*. Winchester: Zero Books.
The Marmot Review (2010) *Post-2010 Strategic Review of Health Inequalities* (The Marmot Review). London: The Marmot Review.
van der Pijl, K. (1984) *The Making of an Atlantic Ruling Class*. London: Verso.
Vygotsky, L. (1934) *Thought and Language*. Cambridge, MA: MIT Press.
Wiley, N. (2004) 'The sociology of inner speech: Saussure meets the dialogical self'. Paper presented at the annual conference of the American Sociology Association. August.
Williams, S. (1999) Is anybody there? Critical realism, chronic illness and the disability debate. *Sociology of Health and Illness* 21: 797–819.
World Health Organization (WHO) (2008) Commission on Social Determinants of Health (CSDH). Closing the Gap in a Generation: Health Equity Through Action on Social Determinants of Health, Geneva: WHO.

9 Deleuze and Guattari

Nick J. Fox

Introduction

Social theorists of health, illness and health care have struggled with a tension between conceptualisations of the body as a biological and as a socially constituted entity, with no end in sight to the capacity of researchers in these two disparate traditions to generate more and more detail about bodies (Fox 2012). The biological sciences have made inroads into the realm of the social, to explain behaviour and social organisation in terms of evolutionary theory and neuroscience (Pitts-Taylor 2010, Tooby and Cosmides 2005). Conversely, social scientists have sometimes regarded biology as irrelevant to the structures and processes of human societies, cultures and economies (Cromby 2004: 798, Turner 1992: 36).

A focus on an exclusively biological or social body is not, however, an option for those whose daily work concerns bodies, amongst others health and social care professionals and the social scientists who research health and illness in the interests of improving patient care and outcomes. Health is an embodied phenomenon that is material, experiential and culturally contextual. For body theorists working to supply a coherent and holistic understanding of embodiment to inform professional health practices and research, it is essential to find a way to explain the dual character of the body, without reducing one or other aspect to a footnote. An intellectually coherent theory that recognises that the body is always both biological and social, and that these aspects of its character together make it what it is, can supply an effective blueprint for the body work of the health and social care professional, and for the experiences of health, illness and care by their patients and clients.

Achieving this balance has not proven to be straightforward. Biological and social scientists start from different places (these days, at the molecular level for the former and at the psychic, cultural or even political level for the latter), and tend to end up with explanations that reflect these starting points. Few academics or professionals have sufficient knowledge and experience of both traditions to move seamlessly between natural and social aspects of embodiment, nor should this be an essential requirement for a holistic insight. In this chapter, I want to introduce a perspective, deriving from the work of Gilles Deleuze, in partnership on occasions with Félix Guattari, which holds substantial promise as a basis for an analysis that can engage with both the biological and physical aspects of embodiment and health on one hand, and the social and cultural on the other, and be comprehensible to both natural and social science traditions.

Relatively ignored in Anglophone sociology until recently, the work of Deleuze and Guattari concerning the connections between body, self and social world offers some interesting ways of thinking about embodiment, and consequently about illness, health and health care. Intrinsic to Deleuze and Guattari's position is the recognition of the link between body, subjectivity and culture. Bodies' physical, psychological and cultural relations, and their capacity to affect and be affected by these relations, are the substrate for embodiment and identity, but also for a radical conception of health as defined by what (else) a body can do. This conception focuses on the body's capacities for engaging with the world around it: physically, psychologically and socially. Sociologists have used Deleuze and Guattari's approach to theorise health, illness and human development (Buchanan 1997, Duff 2010, Fox 2002, 2012, Fox and Ward 2008a), and the perspective offers considerable promise as a means both to develop theoretical understanding of health and illness, and to address the practice and delivery of health care and enhance health and well-being.

In this chapter, I will proceed by summarising the three key elements in Deleuze and Guattari's theoretical position: the *body-without-organs (BwO)*, *assemblages* and *territorialisation*. These abstractions will be explored to suggest how Deleuze and Guattari's conceptions can be used to think creatively about the confluence between the body and the social world, and provide new understanding concerning health and illness. Then, by asking the Deleuzian question 'what can a body do?', I examine how bodily relations and affects (meaning here, the capacity to affect and be affected) mediate 'health' and 'illness', and how these concepts are radicalised by this focus on the body's capacities and potentiality. Finally I will explore some consequences for health care deriving from Deleuze and Guattari's approach.

Deleuze, Guattari and the body

The French philosopher Gilles Deleuze was born in 1925. As a student of philosophy in 1940s Paris, Deleuze's influences included Nietzsche, Bergson, Heidegger and Spinoza. Works including *Difference and Repetition* (1994) and *The Logic of Sense* (1990) established a perspective on the relationship between mind and matter at odds with the 'state philosophy' that proceeded from Plato to Kant and Hegel (Deleuze and Guattari 1988: 376, Massumi 1988: xi). Deleuze's perspective on the body emerged from his reading of Spinoza, set out most extensively in his work *Expressionism in Philosophy: Spinoza* (Deleuze 1992). Here he applied Spinoza's focus on the body's relations and its capacities to affect and be affected, and the key question that follows: what can a body do? He linked this to Artaud's contrast between a medicalised *body-with-organs* with a *body-without-organs* in which biology, culture and identity are confluent (Deleuze and Guattari 1984: 9).

Deleuze established an intellectual partnership with the psychoanalyst Félix Guattari shortly after the May 1968 Paris revolt by students and workers.

Guattari was born in 1930 and following studies in pharmacy and philosophy became involved in oppositional politics, both as a member of the French Communist Party and in challenges to traditional models of mental illness and its treatment. During the 1960s he underwent psychoanalysis with Lacan and subsequently became a Lacanian analyst. However, it was his rejection of Lacan's blend of Freud and Saussurian structuralism, in favour of an effort to synthesise Freud and Marx, which provided the basis for his association with Deleuze (Bogue 1989: 5–6).

The corpus of Deleuze and Guattari's shared authorship includes the major works *Anti-Oedipus* (1984), *A Thousand Plateaus* (1988) and *What is Philosophy?* (1994). In these works, Deleuze's philosophy was applied to the social and political issues of Guattari's anti-psychiatrism, but in so doing gained both immediacy and attraction for social scientists of embodiment and health. For both Deleuze and Guattari, the collaboration over their first joint work, *Anti-Oedipus* (published in France in 1972, and sub-titled *Capitalism and Schizophrenia*), may be seen as synergistic from earlier (though different) commitments and intellectual influences, and as an innovative direction that was to be developed over the following decade. Their collaboration continued into the 1990s: until Guattari's death, which was followed shortly afterwards by Deleuze's own demise.

Deleuze and Guattari's first collaboration, *Anti-Oedipus* (1984), was both an attack on Lacanian psychoanalysis and the formulation of a radical ontology. As materialists, they sought to undermine Lacan's continuation of the Freudian focus on 'desire-as-lack' as the prime motor of psychodynamics. In this corpus, it is the lack or absence of an object (food, the mother, the phallus) translated into the realm of the 'symbolic' that may both lead to neurosis, but also supply the possibility of 'cure' once this symbolic desire is exposed. Deleuze and Guattari deny the latter proposition, arguing that it is only by challenging or changing the physical or psychological relations to *real* things or concepts (as opposed to their psychic symbols) that we may break free from the constraints of the social. They saw capitalism as the source of oppression and repression, in place of Freud's focus on the family and early childhood experiences. Both psychotherapy and progressive political action, they argued, must focus on the material roots of oppression rather than the psychic processes that are oppression's outcome.

Deleuze and Guattari do not deny the existence of a symbolic desire-as-lack, but propose in addition a conception of *positive desire* that is both real and productive, in the sense that it establishes real relations with objects and concepts (Deleuze and Guattari 1988: 254). This desire can be understood as a *creative* affirmation of potential (Massumi 1992: 174) akin to Nietzsche's will-to-power (Bogue 1989: 23–24). By the exertion of this will-to-power, it is possible for humans to be creative rather than reactive, to meet their (real) needs and become free from capitalist oppression.

The importance of Deleuze and Guattari's emphasis on this creative potential is developed in their follow-up work *A Thousand Plateaus* (1988), which focuses less on the ills of psychoanalysis and more on the politics of resistance (Massumi 1992: 82). Deleuze and Guattari develop their understanding of human beings as active and motivated rather than passive and determined, incorporating their engagement with the world through an ongoing work of 'experimentation' (Deleuze and Guattari 1988: 149–51). Embodiment emerges in the dialogical play of social processes and affirmative, creative and *embodied* experimentation/engagement with the world. The *body-without-organs* (BwO) is the locus of this dynamic encounter, *assemblages* of relations establish the limits that comprise the BwO, and *territorialisation* and *deterritorialisation* set out what 'else' a body can do, and the capacities of the body to resist and become.

The body-without-organs

For Deleuze and Guattari, the body does what it does because of the dynamic interaction between two elements. On one hand there are the relations (inward and outward) that a body has with its physical and social context, enabling it to affect and be affected (Fox and Ward 2008a: 1008). On the other, Deleuze and Guattari are keen to recognise an active, experimenting, engaged and engaging body, with the capacity to form new relations, and the desire to do so (Buchanan 1997: 83). This contrasts with deterministic biological or social explanations, which can give the impression that the body is totally 'written' by its genes or by human culture, with little room for any originality. In Deleuze and Guattari's model, the body is creative and engaged both biologically and socially, not a passive vehicle for the environment or the social context to mould. A body can do this and it can do that, in relation to the situations and settings it inhabits, and to its aspirations within an unfolding, active experimentation.

The creative force motivating the body is a feature of all living organisms, according to Deleuze and Guattari (1988: 315). A bacterium, an insect, a bird or a domestic cat are all driven in ways appropriate to their nature: to find food and an environment niche, to find a mate and reproduce, perhaps to care for their offspring. This motivation interacts with the relations to establish the limits of what the insect's or the cat's body can do (its capacities to affect and be affected). 'Hard-wired' instincts drive non-human animals to fulfil their needs for food, shelter and reproduction, though these motivations are mediated through learning and experience to shape each animal's idiosyncratic behaviours. For human beings, things are more complicated (but the dynamic remains the same) because of the extent and diversity of our potential relations, our self-aware reflexivity and our capacity for complex social organisation, economics, politics and culture. We have relations that are proper to our physiology, to our environment, and to our aspirations to talk, to work, to love, to reason or whatever. Humans develop broad (and highly individualised) capacities to affect and be affected by these myriad relations.

Deleuze and Guattari described the body that emerges from this confluence of relations and creative potential as the '*body-without-organs*' (Deleuze and Guattari 1988: 149ff.), often shortened to *BwO*. For them, the important body is not the physical biological entity of biomedicine (they call this 'the organism' or the *body-with-organs*). From the moment of birth – perhaps even before – the BwO is constituted out of this confluence between relations and creative capacity. The BwO of the newborn infant is delimited largely by the drives for food, comfort and warmth. Maturation and experience bring a multiplication of the range of relations, until for an adult human, they are myriad: physical, psychological, emotional and cultural. The discipline of the nursery and the schoolroom, the gendering and sexualisation of adolescence, the routines of work and the growth and disillusionment of ageing progressively create the relations that establish the limits of the body. Indeed, this is the easiest way to understand the BwO, as the limit of what a body can do.

Asssemblages

As I noted earlier, in Deleuze and Guattari's model, the body is not simply 'written' by the environment and the social world, and this is an important point. We know from our own experience that humans do not respond like computers to stimuli, but in complex and sometimes unpredictable ways that suggest an active, motivated engagement with living, the capacity to make choices and act on the world around us. Deleuze and Guattari reject the view that a body's relations (all the physical, psychological and social relations described earlier) directly determine what it can do. Rather the relations contribute to what Deleuze and Guattari (1988: 88) call *assemblages*. These are the outcomes of the interaction between a body's relations and its active motivation. They develop in unpredictable ways 'in a kind of chaotic network of habitual and non-habitual connections, always in flux, always reassembling in different ways' (Potts 2004: 19).

Assemblages are always about process: 'doing' not 'being'. Deleuze and Guattari use the metaphor of a machine to describe how assemblages connect together elements of the body with its relations (Bogue 1989: 91): they argue that every aspect of living, and our experience of the world, contribute to these assemblages. However, within an assemblage

> the relations between bodies, technologies, discourses, regimes of signs and power relations intersect in a manner in which no one term functions as determinant and in which the autonomous specific status of each, as different, in and of themselves, can be accounted for. Dominant relations of power/knowledge are never stable or eternal and as functional elements of an assemblage, they are open to becoming otherwise in shifting fields of connection.
> (Currier 2003: 336)

Assemblages are thus elaborated from disparate elements that can be material, psychic or abstract. For instance, there is an 'eating assemblage', comprising (in no particular order), at least:

mouth–food – energy – appetite

there is a working assemblage comprising, at least:

> body – task–money – career

a sexuality assemblage comprising, at least:

> sex organ – arousal – object of desire

and so forth. The relations can be drawn from any of the domains, material or non-material, but in each case, you will note, the assemblage is dynamic not static: it is about the embodied process of eating or working or sexual desiring, not about a state of being. Furthermore, the assemblage will vary from person to person, contingent on the precise relations that exist as a consequence of experience, beliefs and attitudes, or from bodily predispositions.

Because humans have the capacity for psychological processing and social and cultural interactions, it is virtually impossible for their assemblages to consist merely of biological components. While a newborn infant's eating assemblage may comprise:

> hunger – mouth–food

it is quickly elaborated into

> hunger – mouth–food – nipple – mother.

During childhood it will be further elaborated into

> hunger – mouth–food – appetite – tastes – mother – nipple

with the relations to nipple and mother gradually fading in importance once weaned. For the adult, however, an eating assemblage might comprise:

> hunger – mouth–food – appetite – tastes – money – shopping – dietary choices – time

and many other relations particular to the context and experiences of the individual. A vegetarian's eating assemblage will include a commitment to ethics or ecology, while that of a food allergy sufferer will involve not only a negative relation to nuts, dairy products or whatever, but also the experience of an allergic reaction. Both have emerged from an infantile relation to food, but in very different directions. These differences explain why the embodiment of one person differs from another.

We can use this model of assemblages to explore embodiment, including processes associated with health and illness (Fox and Ward 2008a). A general health care assemblage might comprise

> patient – disease – doctor – biomedicine – health technology.

There is an assemblage with particular significance for the anorexic or the dieter comprising:

> mouth – food – body shape – control (Fox et al. 2005b).

Potts (2004: 22) describes an impotence treatment assemblage comprising:

> Viagra or other pharmaceuticals – erectile dysfunction – medicalisation – partners – doctors – Viagra-fied penis.

People's responses to health care are explained by the idiosyncrasies of their own particular health care assemblage.

It is the totality of assemblages that creates the BwO and thereby the conditions of possibility for the body. Assemblages link the individual's body to the social and natural environments (Bogue 1989: 91), creating the substrate that both defines a person's capacities and her/his limits. As a consequence, bodies should be understood as

> neither fixed nor given, but as particular historical configurations of the material and immaterial, captured and articulated through various assemblages which to some extent determine them as particular bodies, but never manage entirely to exclude the movement of differing and the possibility of becoming otherwise.
>
> (Currier 2003: 332)

> In a sense, the body is lived through the assemblages, which as noted earlier, are always processual: they are about doing, not being. Unpacking an individual's assemblages can enable understanding of how a person may respond to her/his environment, her/his experiences of illness and healthcare, and may be the basis for therapy or support.
>
> (Fox and Ward 2008a)

Territories of the body

The discussion so far of the relations that a body has with its context has focused on the quantity and the diversity of its relations, and left to one side any thought about the qualities and characteristics of the relations themselves. So a body may have a physical relation to gravity, a psychological relation to its parent, and a cultural relation to a nationality. In each case, behind the relation, there is a force (strong or weak) at work. Gravity acts on the physical body to constrain its movement, the parent acts psychologically as a force over behaviour and attitudes that may weaken over time as a body moves from child to adulthood. Nationality is a force affecting an embodied sense of identity and perhaps a choice of partners or associates. Each body has its own relations, but in all cases these relations bring to bear forces, pushing or pulling the body (more properly, the BwO) in one direction or another (Duff 2010: 625).

It follows that the BwO (comprised of assemblages of relations) is a *territory* constantly contested and fought over by rival forces. The assemblages of relations determine the overall shape, intensity and direction of the consequent vector of forces. Importantly, in Deleuze and Guattari's approach, once again there is no need to differentiate the realm from which a force derives: physical, psychological and social forces can all be treated together. An eating assemblage might include physical resources (scarcity or plenty of specific foods), psychological preferences and tastes, and cultural restrictions such as kosher requirements. A vegetarian eating assemblage will include physical, psychological, social and philosophical and ethical relations, with their associated forces (Fox and Ward 2008b: 2587). The outcome vector of these disparate forces limits the body to a vegetarian diet, except perhaps in circumstances where hunger becomes more dominant than ethical attachments, in which case the assemblage will modify, altering the body's affects regarding meat and its ethical principles.

So the BwO is the target of what Deleuze and Guattari call *territorialisation* (Deleuze and Guattari 1994: 67ff.). The consequence may be a change in character or a redefinition. Thus the force of the sun's gravity territorialises the earth as it travels through space, acting on it through the exertion of a force, and turning it into a 'satellite'. Biomedicine territorialises an individual consulting a health professional, transforming her/him into a patient, and her/his symptoms into a disease. It follows that many aspects of human interaction involve territorialisation, with one or both parties affected. Territories and territorialisations are often concerned with socially created meanings: philosophy and ideology have historically territorialised land as 'nations', homeland or fatherland (Deleuze and Guattari 1994: 68).

However, all forces may be resisted. The earth does not succumb entirely to the sun's gravitational pull, because its velocity through space acts as a counterforce that always seeks to escape the sun, and move away on its own trajectory. The resultant orbit is the vector of force and counterforce. Because forces add and subtract from each other, it is possible for one force to *deterritorialise* a territorialised BwO. It is also possible for another force to then *reterritorialise* the BwO again. The BwO is thus both the site where the body's relations territorialise it, but also the site of resistance and refusal. In this way, the BwO is constructed and reconstructed (territorialised) continually, as forces interact within the assemblages. For example, an individual consulting a health professional may resist and refuse the patient role, and find an alternative embodiment, such as a 'consumer' of health services (Fox *et al.* 2005).

As a model of embodiment, territorialisation provides an explanatory framework for how the forces of the social impinge on individuals or cultures, from class, gender and ethnic stratification through to the creation of subjectivities in people as, for instance, 'women', 'husbands', 'patients' and 'risk takers'. However, Deleuze and Guattari also assert the capacity of the body to resist (and thus shift the balance of) these forces, either by application of cultural, economic or physical resources, or with outside assistance. While physical forces may be overcome only through training or with the aid of technology (a Scuba suit will allow a human body to breathe under water), most social territorialisations involve some act of interpretation, so there are endless possibilities for de- and reterritorialisation through a body's cognitive capacities. Language offers the potential for humans to interpret the world with infinite variety: we all indulge in cognitive behavioural therapy endlessly! Where forces are too strong to resist in this way, outside help by a friend, another citizen or a caring professional may offer the necessary counterbalance to oppression (Fox 1999: 77ff.).

Having looked at the fundamental building blocks in Deleuze and Guattari's model, I will now explore how their approach can be used to supply new understandings of health and illness. I start with Deleuze and Guattari's critique of biomedicine and the 'body-with-organs'.

The body-*with*-organs, and beyond

One territorialisation that is of particular relevance for those engaged in health care is the establishment of the biomedical body. The body-*with*-organs is the name that Deleuze and Guattari gave to this biological body, which they also call the 'organism' (Deleuze and Guattari 1988: 158). The body-with-organs is the product of powerful forces emanating from biomedicine, and inherent in the medicalising processes of health care that turn bodies into patients, and their experiences of their sick bodies into case histories of disease. The sick, the convalescent, the disabled are all part of this territorialisation: the history of health has been written, and continues to be written within this territory (cf. Foucault 1976).

Deleuze and Guattari's model of the body suggests that the body-*with*-organs is only one territorialisation of the body among many. Social science models of the body (and of health) are rival territorialisations, which seek to show how social and cultural forces construct our bodies. While it is unquestionable that bodies are the subjects of physical and biological forces, the point about the body-*with*-organs or 'the organism' is that it has become a very powerful model of the body, to the extent that it can be hard to imagine an alternative, particularly when the subject of this territorialisation is sick, vulnerable and dependent on health professionals who use this model of the body to inform their work and their interactions with patients (Kleinman 1988).

Using Deleuze and Guattari's model, we can understand the 'patient' and her/his health/illness in terms of the relations, forces and assemblages that construct her/his BwO: the limit of what their bodies can do. In the case of a BwO that is also the body-*with*-organs, this is a body fully defined by biomedicine. Part of Deleuze and Guattari's project was to undermine any dominant territorialisations, including the body-*with*-organs (Deleuze and Guattari 1988: 24). They wanted to show how it is possible to resist territorialisation, to establish what they called a *line of flight* from that territorialisation to a new embodiment (Deleuze and Guattari 1988: 55). While the new embodiment (or BwO) after a line of flight also involves a reterritorialisation, it may be one where a body can do more (or different things) than it could do in its previous territorialisation. Often the deterritorialisation is momentary and perhaps inconsequential: the BwO moves just a little from its previous position before reterritorializing in a new patterning. At other times, it may be substantial and life changing, a line of flight that carries the BwO into unimagined realms of possibility and 'nomadic' becoming-other (Deleuze and Guattari 1988: 24).

Deleuze and Guattari saw themselves very much on the side of deterritorialisation and resistance. In relation to mental health, they called this process 'schizoanalysis' (Deleuze and Guattari 1984: 273); more generally as a strategy for living, they called it 'nomadology' (Deleuze and Guattari 1988: 23). Nomadology must be thought of not as an outcome but as a process, as a line of flight that continually resists the sedentary, the single fixed perspective (Deleuze and Guattari 1988: 381). A commitment to deterritorialisation and the nomad is intrinsically political, always on the side of freedom, experimentation and becoming, always opposed to power, territory and the fixing of identity (ibid: 24).

Deleuze and Guattari's conception of the nomad is pregnant with significance for our understanding of the social character of health, illness and health care, and also for a practical resistance to biomedicine. Biomedicine has achieved hegemony for the body-with-organs: the 'organism'. Deleuze and Guattari demonstrated a similar territorialisation of mental health and illness in the individualisation and familialisation of pathology, and posed their 'schizoanalysis' as a nomadic alternative in *Anti-Oedipus*. Unlike some other social analyses of health care, which are pessimistic about resisting the dominant discourses around health and illness, Deleuze and Guattari offer a perspective that has great promise for radicalising the theory and practice of health care. What if there were to be a nomadological refusal of the territory of 'health' itself?

Applying the model: what can a body do?

To begin to explore how Deleuze and Guattari's perspective can help to shed new light on health and illness, and develop health care practice, I will turn to the key question that Deleuzianism asks about bodies. Deleuze drew heavily upon Spinoza's philosophy in developing his perspective on the body (Duff 2010: 624). Rather than considering what a body *is*, students of embodiment in the natural and social scientists should ask: *what can a body do?* This question is

> the critical means of finding out what masochists, drug users, obsessives and paranoiacs are actually trying to do. The question works by staking out an area of *what* a body actually can do. This area is restricted by obvious physical constraints which must be respected. But this does not mean that there is no beyond, or that a beyond cannot be desired. And it is just this *beyond* – beyond the physical limits of the physical body – that the concept of the body-without-organs articulates … It is the body's limits that define the BwO, not the other way around.
>
> (Buchanan 1997: 79, his emphases)

Note that this approach is not functionalistic, indeed it rejects efforts to define the essential nature of a body. Deleuze and Guattari's approach consists not in assessing bodily cause and effect (it has kidneys, so it can excrete), but in counting a body's *relations* and its *affects* (its capacity to affect and be affected) (Deleuze and Guattari 1988: 257), which may be many or few. Asking 'what can a body do?' recognises an active, experimenting, engaged and engaging body, not one passively written in systems of thought. Bodies are not the locus at which forces act, they are the production of the interactions of forces. A body is *the capacity to form new relations, and the desire to do so.* (Buchanan 1997: 83).

Asking a body, what it can do (which are its relations?) informs us about its BwO (the confluences of a body with its affects and relations), about assemblages of relations, about deterritorialisation and lines of flight (the trajectories that open up possibilities for becoming-other). Counting the relations ('natural' or 'cultural' – these terms become meaningless) and affects of a body can indicate how it is territorialised; fostering new relations may open the way to a line of flight. The uniqueness of individual bodies lies in their diverse relations and affects (Duff 2010: 625). This provides a methodology for exploring bodies that has been exploited by social scientists (Duff 2010, Fox and Ward 2008a).

Let us ask this question about the human body in illness and health. Buchanan (1997) focused on some BwOs that are congruent with the Deleuze and Guattari project: the anorexic body, the paralysed body, the schizoid body (Buchanan 1997: 8ff.), just as Deleuze and Guattari (1988: 150) considered the hypochondriac, drugged and masochistic bodies. In my own essay (Fox 2002), I looked at some less extreme BwOs, to map the limits of 'healthy' and 'sick' bodies. Here I will focus on the assemblages (and their constituent relations) that constitute certain bodies-without-organs.

The contagious assemblage

The body reaches out to others to make it like itself; it does this on behalf of the bacterium, however much it tries not to do so. It has relations to the body that infected it, and so to all the bodies in the epidemic, and it stands in a one-to-many relation to all those it will infect. It is a pariah body, its relations do not wish it as a relation.

The neoplastic assemblage

The body has relations to itself and to the neoplasia within, to the health professions, to therapies, to life and death, to (fear of) the future. It subjects itself to censorship, to moralistic outrage. It appraises itself: 'this part is good, it can remain; this part is bad, it must be excised or burnt or poisoned or overcome by positive mental effort'. The body is conservative, it is suspicious of novelty, of otherness: it is a control freak because the worst consequence is to lose control.

The weight-loss assemblage

The body enhances, concentrates and strengthens its relation with food, it thinks of everything it sees: 'I can consume you, you can become part of me'. Life is measured in kilograms and days: the body becomes utopian, Puritan and millenarian, imagining a time and a remade slim body, which has yet to come into existence but which once attained will be free of pain and longing, gloriously released from the shackles of unconsummated desire.

The hypochondriac assemblage

This body has been consumed by the diseases it fears. There is nothing left, it has been burnt out, it has become pathology. The BwO rattles, like an empty husk whose only contents are the ailments that began this hopeless territorialisation.

We can thus make sense of the 'patient' and their health/illness in terms of the relations, affects and assemblages that set the limit of what the body can do. This is not, however, an exercise in assessing mobility or capacity to work or to reason or whatever. What a body can do is not a matter of health assessment or pathology diagnosis, but of its capacity to enter into relations with other bodies, to become-other (Duff 2010: 625). Assemblages territorialise the body by limiting its affects. Buchanan offers the example of the anorexic (the 'slimming body' gone critical, perhaps), who

> endeavours to obtain freedom, to become free, via the pathway of an intensive hunger, eliminating in the process all extensive demand (demands of the body-organism). Hunger that is not determined by the demands of the body is intense because it is now for itself; as such, it would be more correct to describe it as 'hungering' not hunger. The problem for the anorexic, however, and this is the inherent danger of all self-motivated becoming, is that far from accelerating becoming, what he or she actually does is deform it. Intensifying a particular (affect is) ... a gross delimitation of becoming itself. It confuses the blissfully passive beyond of becoming which Nietzsche idealizes, with the passivity of the already become.
>
> (Buchanan 1997: 87)

A body (BwO) that has become (rather than being in the process of becoming) has suffered territorialisation, into a territory that may not easily be escaped. The valetudinarian has become an invalid, the dementing body loses all sense of continuity. For some people, being a 'patient' or receiving care is just such a reterritorialisation, one that closes down possibilities, creating a body-self trammelled by dependency. Having become, there is no becoming left to do. Singularity of purpose leads not to transcendence, but to death (Deleuze and Guattari 1988: 149).

Becoming other requires the multiplication of affects, not the intensification of a single affect or relation. It is an opening-up to difference, to possibility and to the 'rightness' of the many rather than the few or the one (Deleuze and Guattari

1988: 24–25). This is not an easy conclusion to draw: multiplication of affects and relations, particularly if one's resources are limited, may not be something that can be achieved independently: we may need all the help we can get. There is an agenda here that goes beyond the clinic and the academy and encompasses health and social policy, economics and the politics of welfare. But it can also be applied to the most practical aspects of health care when professionals' work opens up possibilities for patients and clients (Fox 1999: 85ff.).

To give two simple examples: a patient's BwO (territorialised by biomedicine, by pain and by fear) may be deterritorialised by a health care worker or friend who treats them as something more than a collection of pathologies; a child's BwO may be deterritorialised (and reterritorialised) by the adult who treats her as an equal (Fox 1999: 89). By encouraging patients to pursue an aspiration, it may open locked doors onto new vistas (Buchanan 1997: 85). Importantly, this

> does not result in the patient being restored to his or her former self, rather, using the newly awakened affect, he or she is encouraged to invent a new self.
> (Buchanan 1997: 85)

This is important for health care professionals, as they, and the care they provide, can be the relation that may either deterritorialise a person or patient, helping them to move beyond the current limits of their embodiment, or reterritorialise them, typically by defining them narrowly in biomedical terms (Fox 1993: 84ff.). Care can be an invaluable resource to enable a line of flight from the physical and psychological limits of a chronic illness or disability.

Deleuze and Guattari and 'health'

What, however, of the body in health? If there is an ill-health assemblage and a sickening body, is there also a *health assemblage*, and a becoming-healthy body? Can the approach to embodiment that looks at relations, affects and assemblages help to make sense of the BwO of health?

When looking at health and illness, it is the interplay of relations with the active, engaging, becoming-other motivation of the body that determines whether a body (or BwO) is 'healthy' or 'sick'. In Buchanan's (1997) essay on Deleuze, he appropriates the term 'health' as a metaphor for the body's capacity to form relations, regardless of whether they are actually associated with a traditional, narrow sense of health (Buchanan 1997: 82, and cf. Fox 1993 on 'arché-health'). His broader definition, however, can be happily narrowed to the confines of health care for the purposes of this chapter. Within such narrowed limits, we can assert that, from a Deleuzian perspective, it is the capacity of the body to form relations that determines its sickness or health: its capacities to affect and be affected (Buchanan 1997: 80).

It follows that 'health' is not just an absence of disease relations (as suggested in the biomedical model), but the opposite: the proliferation of a body's capacities to affect and be affected. Illness closes down these capacities, health is defined in terms of the body's widened capacities to make, resist and transform its relations. These capacities include the body's biological functions, its psychological well-being and the social and cultural 'capital' it can draw upon. Friends, family and health professionals may be important in enhancing these capacities, tipping the balance towards health by providing physical, psychological, economic or sociocultural support and encouragement. The 'health' of a body is influenced by

> ... refracted and resisted relations, biological capabilities or cultural mind-sets, alliances with friends or health workers, struggles for control over treatment or conditions of living. Health is neither an absolute... to be aspired towards, nor an idealised outcome of 'mind-over-matter'. It is a process of becoming by (the body), of rallying relations, resisting physical or social territorialisation, and experimenting with what is, and what it might become.
> (Fox 2002: 360)

Health is never a final outcome in this Deleuzian perspective. Rather it is a process, a becoming-other that fluctuates along with the body's capacities. The BwO marks the limits of what (else) a body can do, but this is always in flux, always becoming other. So we should never look for a static embodiment of health or illness, rather what we should seek is the ongoing becoming-other of the body. Rather than saying a body is healthy, we might talk about its 'becoming healthy', or about the 'healthing' of a body, to remind us of the active processes involved and the fluctuating nature of embodied health. This approach reminds us of the continually changing process of embodiment and the complex mix of relations that contribute to health.

Buchanan's (1997) appropriation of 'health' to describe a much wider conception of bodily well-being, and Fox's (1993) introduction of 'arché-health' as a concept to describe a deterritorialising becoming-other of the body, both recall that well-being extends far beyond the confines set by biomedicine. The Deleuzian model of embodiment and what a body can do has been applied by sociologists to address a number of broader aspects of bodies. Fox (2005) examined the biological, psychological and cultural relations that influence what an ageing body can do, exploring the combinations of relations that make ageing an individual experience. Potts (2004) has explored how new pharmaceutical technologies such as Viagra that apparently enhance a body's capacities may in fact limit what a body can do, with consequences both for those using the technology and those around them. Fox and Ward (2008a) have used a Deleuzian approach to explore health identities: the assemblages that shape how people respond to health, illness and health care. They looked at a range of health identities, from a traditional patient through to a resisting consumer. By exploring the relations that bodies have – an approach that Deleuze called 'ethology' (Duff 2010: 625) – a person's health identity can be explored empirically. Duff (2010) argues that this kind of ethological approach may be used more widely, to explore human development from cradle to grave, in the 'five developmental domains of social, cognitive, emotional, material and moral development' (Duff 2010: 629). Development over the life course can be seen as a gradual enhancement of a body's 'force of existing' or power of acting (ibid: 630). For Currier (2003), Deleuze and Guattari's conception of assemblages offers a radical way to understand patriarchy and how feminism may challenge masculine power relations. In my view, these studies scratch the surface of a broader project to rethink bodies in health and illness, both theoretically and practically in day-to-day health and social care.

Conclusions

In this chapter I have set out the key elements of Deleuze and Guattari's model of the body, and shown how these can be applied to provide new understandings of health, illness and health care.

The first important aspect to Deleuze and Guattari's model concerns the character of embodiment. An advantage of their approach is that it does not privilege biology or social aspects of the body. The body is clearly both biological and a cultural product, and by focusing not on what a body is, but what relations a body has with the physical, psychological and cultural environment that surrounds it, we are released from a nature/culture dualism. Similarly a body's affects (what it can affect and be affected by) derive from all and any of these domains, and we need not set culture over biology or *vice versa*. Relations and affects from different domains interact to constitute the body-without-organs (BwO), and assemblages link together elements from physical and cultural domains. The BwO is the limit of what a body can do, not in a functionalist sense, but in terms of its relations and the play of forces of those relations. For patients, people with disabilities, older adults and for anyone, the social and the natural worlds may impinge to territorialise the BwO, to establish limits from which it is hard to escape. The BwO emerges from the multiplicity of physical, psychological and social relations of a body, combining in unique ways that are always in flux.

The second element of Deleuze and Guattari's model emphasises that embodiment is not the passive outcome of 'inscription' by these various relations, but a dynamic, reflexive, 'reading' of the social by an active, motivated human being. For Deleuze and Guattari, the BwO is like an uncharted territory, but one whose possession must be fought over, inch by inch. The BwO is endlessly territorialised, deterritorialised and reterritorialised. Territorialisation is a function both of the forces of the physical and social world, and by the motivated, 'experimenting' BwO as it becomes other. Territorialisations are resisted and subverted by the experimenting, 'experiencing' body, conjuring the endless permutations of living: of health, illness, sexual desire, ageing and death; the multiplying, becoming-other body that is always capable of a new interpretation, another nuance.

Finally, we may understand 'health' as the body's capacity to affect and be affected, and thus its *resistance* to forces of territorialisation that limit these capacities. Resistance is not only a possibility: it is the creative force of the body that refracts the physical and biological, psychological or emotional, social and cultural relations that impinge upon it. The 'health' of a body is the outcome of biological capabilities and cultural mind-sets, alliances with friends or health workers, struggles for control over treatment or conditions of living. It is neither an absolute (defined by whatever discipline) to be aspired towards, nor an idealised outcome of 'mind-over-matter'. It is a process of becoming, of rallying capacities, resisting physical or social territorialisation, and experimenting with what is, and what might become.

This perspective makes health and health care intrinsically political. For 'patients' and for everyone, the politics of health and illness are about engaging with the real struggles of people as they are territorialised – by biology *or* by culture, as they resist, and as they encourage others in their aspirations, development and lives. Health is processual, and both at the level of the individual and the wider public health, this is a process that encompasses natural and social science disciplines. For health care (as for education, citizenship and every aspect of social action), the analysis developed from the work of Deleuze and Guattari suggests an agenda for its practitioners that fosters deterritorialisation in the bodies of those for whom they care (Fox 1995, 1999), and generates a politics of health that transcends economic and management perspectives. To engage productively with such agendas collapses disciplinary boundaries and establishes a pressing need for collaboration between medical and caring professions, social and political scientists, social activists, indeed everyone with a body.

References

Bogue, R. (1989) *Deleuze and Guattari*. London: Routledge.
Buchanan, I. (1997) The problem of the body in Deleuze and Guattari, or, what can a body do? *Body & Society*, 3, 73–91.
Cromby, J. (2004) Between constructionism and neuroscience: the societal co-constitution of embodied subjectivity. *Theory and Psychology*, 14(6), 797–821.
Currier, D. (2003) Feminist technological futures: Deleuze and body/technology assemblages, *Feminist Theory*, 4(3), 321–38.
Deleuze, G. (1990) *The Logic of Sense*. New York: Columbia University Press.
——(1992) *Expressionism in Philosophy: Spinoza*. New York: Zone Books.
——(1994) *Difference and Repetition*. London: Athlone.
Deleuze, G. and Guattari, F. (1984) *Anti-Oedipus: Capitalism and Schizophrenia*. London: Athlone.
——(1988) *A Thousand Plateaus*. London: Athlone.
——(1994) *What is Philosophy?* London: Verso.
Duff, C. (2010) Towards a developmental ethology: exploring Deleuze's contribution to the study of health and human development. *Health*, 14(6), 619–34.
Foucault, M. (1976) *The Birth of the Clinic*. London: Tavistock.
Fox, N. J. (1993) *Postmodernism, Sociology and Health*. Buckingham: Open University Press.
——(1995) Postmodern perspectives on care: the Vigil and the Gift. *Critical Social Policy*, 15, 107–24.
——(1999) *Beyond Health. Postmodernism and Embodiment*. London: Free Association Books.
——(2002) Refracting health: Deleuze, Guattari and body/self. *Health*, 6(1), 347–64.
——(2005) Cultures of ageing in Thailand and Australia (What can an ageing body do?). *Sociology*, 39(3), 501–18.
——(2012) *The Body*. Cambridge: Polity Press.
Fox, N. J. and Ward, K. J. (2008a) 'What are health identities and how may we study them?' *Sociology of Health and Illness*, 30(7), 461–79.

——(2008b) 'You are what you eat? Vegetarians, health and identity'. *Social Science and Medicine*, 66(12): 2585–95.

Fox, N. J., Ward, K. J. and O'Rourke, A. J. (2005) 'Expert patients', pharmaceuticals and the medical model of disease: The case of weight loss, drugs and the Internet. *Social Science and Medicine*, 60(6), 1299–309.

Kleinman, A. (1988) *The Illness Narratives*. New York: Basic Books.

Massumi, B. (1988) Translators's foreword. In Deleuze, G. and Guattari, F. *A Thousand Plateaus*. London: Athlone.

——(1992) *A Users Guide to Capitalism and Schizophrenia*. Cambridge, MA: MIT Press.

Pitts-Taylor, V. (2010) The plastic brain; neoliberalism and the neuronal self. *Health*, 14(6), 625–52.

Potts, A. (2004) Deleuze on Viagra (Or, what can a Viagra-body do?). *Body 36*.

Tooby, J. and Cosmides, L. (2005) Conceptual foundations of evolutionary psychology. In D. M. Buss (ed.) *The Handbook of Evolutionary Psychology* (pp. 5–67). Hoboken, NJ: Wiley.

Turner, B. (1992) *Regulating Bodies*. London: Routledge.

10 Health and medicine in the information age

Castells, informational capitalism and the network society

Simon J. Williams

Introduction

It is perhaps inevitable, in writing a chapter for this second edition, that I found myself reaching for the first edition and leafing back through my chapter on Goffman's sociological theory of stigma and its applications to health and illness. In doing so, despite important developments in the intervening time period on the structural and political dimensions of stigma (Scambler 2009; Monaghan and Williams in press) I am inevitably struck by the contrast between the more micro-oriented sociological concerns pursued therein and the more macro-oriented sociological concerns I shall pursue in this chapter on the sociologist Manuel Castells.

Someone smarter than me no doubt might explore the convergences and micro–macro connections here through a new sociological theory of stigma in the information age and the network society perhaps. My focus, however, will be somewhat different, if not novel, given that my chosen application of Castells to the health domain pertains not to stigma but to sleep. Sleep is an odd choice you may think, particularly for sociology, but it is one that I hope to convince you, the reader, is a befitting example and novel illustration by the end of the chapter.

So why then, of all sociological theorists dead or alive today, have I chosen Castells? And why, for that matter, have I chosen sleep to apply his work to? The short answer to the latter question is not simply that sleep is a novel yet important and fast-growing sociological topic area, but that it's an issue I have been researching for well over a decade now and so, on both theoretical and practical counts, it seemed like a good test case to try out and see. As for the former question, there are two short answers. First, my growing interest in another rich new area of research, namely sociological engagements with the neurosciences, led me to Castells' work given his recent attempts to deepen or enrich his theory of 'communication power' in the network society through recourse to various strands of neuroscience, affective intelligence and political communication theory (of which more below). Second, it seemed inevitable, given my longstanding interests in the media–health nexus, and my growing sociological interests in networks and complexity theory, that sooner or later I would get to reading Castells: the sociological theorist *par excellence* of the information age and the network society.

Two further points are perhaps worth flagging at the outset. First, my reading and hence account of Castells' work will primarily be based on his three-volume study of *The Information Age* and his more recent book *Communication Power*, which consolidates and extends this previous information trilogy in significant new ways. Whilst this seems justified, given Castells is probably best known for this three-volume study, if not the latter more recent book, it should nonetheless be noted that Castells has written over 20 books to date. Others, second, have done a far better job than I can hope to, in the scope of one short chapter, to explore and appraise Castells' work – see for example Stalder (2006); Webster (2002); Webster and Dimitriou (2004). Viewed in this light then, the chapter is best read perhaps as an invitation of sorts for those who wish to go further in terms of both these primary and secondary sources and their potential applications to the health domain.

To date however, to the best of my knowledge, there has been precious little, if any, direct engagement with Castells' work in medical sociology. This indeed is all the more curious when one considers: (i) advances made since the first edition of this volume was published in exploring and linking sociological theory and medical sociology, including a new *Social Theory and Health* journal; and (ii) the significant and growing sociological interest in the media–health nexus and associated issues to do with the role of information and communication technologies (ICTs) in e-health and tele- or virtual medicine today.

What then does Castells have to say about the nature and dynamics of society today, and how might these insights be applied to health? It is to these very issues that we now turn, starting with a brief background biographical sketch of Castells' intellectual debts and departure points.

Intellectual debts and departures: from Marxism to …

Castells was born in 1942 in Hellin, Spain, but grew up mainly in Barcelona at a time when Franco ruled Spain. This no doubt contributed to Castells' early political activism and his abiding interest in urban questions and the city. As a political refugee in Paris by the tender age of 20, Castells completed his Master's degree in law and economics, followed by a doctorate in sociology at the Sorbonne under the supervision of Alain Touraine, and a subsequent post as assistant professor in sociology at the University of Paris in the late 1960s. This was a time, of course, of considerable political struggle and student protest, which Castells, in characteristic fashion, fully immersed himself in. It resulted in Castells' temporary expulsion from France in 1968 and his subsequent reinstatement (thanks to Touraine's efforts) at the *Ecolé de Hautes en Science Sociales* in Paris in 1970 where, as Stalder (2006) notes, he became a leading figure of the new Marxist urban sociology before leaving Paris in 1979 to take up the post of professor of sociology and of city and regional planning at the University of California Berkeley, a post he occupied until 2003. Since then Castells' main academic posts have been as professor and Wallis Annenberg Chair Professor of Communication Technology and Society at the Annenberg School of Communication, University of Southern California, Los

Angeles, and research professor (director of the Internet Interdisciplinary Institute) at the Open University of Catalonia (UoC) in Barcelona.

He has also received numerous awards, honours and accolades, including 14 honorary doctorates, knighthoods by France, Catalonia, Finland, Chile, and Portugal, and various other roles such as adviser in 1992 to Yeltsin on political economic policy, and (founding) member of the European Research Council (European Commission).

Perhaps more importantly for our purposes is the intellectual distance Castells has travelled during this time period, from his early neo-Marxist allegiances and attempts to develop a new Marxist urban sociology (Castells 1978, 1977), to his current concerns and preoccupations with *informationalism* and *communication power* in the *network society* (e.g. Castells 1989, 2000a, 2001, 2009, 2010a, 2010b). It is a journey that has resulted not simply in the abandonment of structural Marxism as a dominant theoretical framework – particularly Castells' early intellectual debts to Althusser – but in a radically revised or redefined role for theory of any kind in his work.

This new role for theory is perhaps worth elaborating on a little further here at the outset, given the concerns of this volume as a whole. Ultimately, we might say, Castells seems more concerned with theory in the service of empirical research than grand theoretical gestures or pretensions. Castells' position, in this regard, might perhaps be characterised as something of a 'pragmatic' approach to theory and a studied indifference to what has gone before in terms of situating his work in relation to past or present sociological theory. He is not interested, in other words, in writing 'books about books' (Castells 2009: 6), nor to fell more rainforests in order to do so, but simply to test his own hypotheses empirically against the vast body of primary and secondary source data he, or perhaps more correctly his students and researchers, have at their disposal.

This of course is not to suggest that Castells is a narrow empiricist: far from it. It is however to suggest that theory and the concepts it generates is, for Castells, a largely disposable or at the very least an eminently revisable tool – i.e. an approach, that is to say, which regards 'theory as a tool box to understand social reality' (Castells 2009: 6) – which by virtue of this very fact can never be complete or comprehensive. Contra Marx moreover, the task in the twenty-first century, Castells declares, is to *interpret* the world differently. Castells' approach in this regard, as Stalder (2006: 40) comments, is perhaps most closely allied to Weber's neo-Kantian position than to Marx in the sense that concepts, at one and the same time, *precede* empirical observation yet can and have to be revised in the light of empirical observations. Reflexive questions regarding both the production and problematisation of his own position, nonetheless, are largely absent in Castells' work – a point I shall return to later when appraising Castells.

It is therefore against this biographical and intellectual backdrop that some of the core sociological themes and concerns of Castells' more recent work on 'communication power' in the 'information age' and the 'network society' must be judged, a key element of which we now turn to.

The network society: dimensions and dynamics

Production: technology, informational capitalism and social change

Technology of course, particularly information and communication technology, is critical to Castells' work since the 1980s, taking relations between technological developments, social dynamics and changing social forms or morphologies as his major problematic.

Although very much a stand-alone or independent contribution with few professed intellectual debts, Castells' work in this respect coincides with an upsurge of other work within the social sciences and humanities in recent decades, which has sought to examine the *social dimensions* and the *social dynamics* of science and technology in society, and the *increasingly technosocial* world we live in these days – see Hackett *et al.* (2007), for example.

How then does Castells conceive of this relationship between technology and social change, particularly in light of his previous structural–Marxist sympathies and Althusserian debts? The simple answer is that technology, Castells stresses, plays a fundamental role in shaping the structural forces of the economy. We might, on this count, take an instructive step back to Bell's famous thesis on *The Coming of Post-industrial Society*, published in 1973, which hinged on the transition from an industrial (manufactured) 'goods' producing society to a more 'service' based post-industrial society. Castells' approach in this regard can be read, on the one hand, as displaying certain affinities with Bell's thesis whilst also, on the other hand, providing a more or less comprehensive corrective or update on it given: (i) the transition from industry to services (as Bell and his followers envisaged) has been far from clear-cut; and (ii) Castells' greater emphasis, as Stalder (2006: 45) comments, on the changing *spatial* organisation of production rather than the changing composition of the labour force. At stake here, in short, is a transition from the industrial age to the *information age*, which has profoundly reconfigured the *spatial* and *temporal* dimensions and dynamics of society.

Expressive of his Marxist roots, Castells also draws a distinction here, in *Volume I* of *The Information Age*, between the *'mode of production'* and the *'mode of development'*. The mode of development, he states, concerns the *'technological arrangements through which labour works on matter to generate the product'* (Castells 2000a: 16, my emphasis). The mode of production, in contrast, captures the *social relations* that make up the economy, or who in other words appropriates the surplus value, as in say capitalism or statism. It is essential for the understanding of social dynamics, Castells argues, to 'maintain the analytical distance and empirical interrelation between modes of production (capitalism, statism) and modes of development (industrial, informational)' (Castells 2000a: 14). Compared to previous modes of development furthermore, the source of productivity in the informational mode of development 'lies in the technology of knowledge generation, information processing, and symbolic communication'. What is distinctive or specific to the new mode of development, in other words, is:

> ... the *action of knowledge upon knowledge itself* as the main source of productivity ... information processing is focussed on improving the technology of information processing as a source of productivity ... informationalism is oriented towards technological development, that is toward the accumulation of knowledge and towards higher levels of complexity in information processing.
> (Castells 2000a: 17, my emphasis)

This then provides the basis for Castells' claims – tied to this significant new phase of capitalist restructuring since the 1980s – that a new 'techno-economic system' is now evident in the form of *'informational capitalism'* (Castells 2000a: 18–19): a system, that is to say, indebted to new information technologies, characterised and organised by technological innovation and centred around *flexibility* and *adaptability*. Without this new information technology indeed, Castells claims, global capitalism would have been a 'much-limited reality, flexible management would have been reduced to labour trimming, and the new round of both capital goods and new consumer products would not have been sufficient to compensate for the reduction in public spending' (Castells 2000a: 19). Thus informationalism is linked to the *'expansion* and *rejuvenation* of capitalism, as industrialism was linked to its constitution as a mode of production' (Castells 2000a: 19, my emphasis). Within this new economy moreover, a premium is placed on flexible, adaptable *'self-programmable'* flows of labour able to 'autonomously process information into specific knowledge' vis-à-vis *'generic workers'* who must be 'ready to adapt to the needs of this new economy or else face displacement by machines or alternative labour forces' (Castells 2009: 33).

Whilst capitalism's restructuring and the diffusion of informationalism, on this reading, were 'inseparable processes on a global scale', Castells (2000a: 20) is also quick to emphasise that 'societies did act/react differently to such processes, according to the specificity of their history, culture, and institutions'. Reference to an 'informational society' therefore may be improper if this implies homogeneity of social forms. One could nevertheless, Castells ventures, justifiably speak here of 'an informational society' in the same way as people talk of an 'industrial society', albeit with two important riders or provisos: 'on the one hand, informational societies, as they currently exist, are capitalist (unlike industrial societies, some of which are statist[1]); on the other hand, we must stress the cultural and institutional diversity of informational societies' (Castells 2000a: 20). All societies then, as this suggests, are affected by capitalism and informationalism in one way or another, with 'many societies (certainly all major societies) already informational, although of different kinds, in different settings, and with specific cultural/institutional expressions' (Castells 2000a: 20–21).

So far so good perhaps, but questions of *determinism* inevitably arise here in all this talk of modes of development and modes of production. This is something we shall return to and deal with more fully later on. Two key points are worth stressing at this point however. First, Castells emphasises the *'relative autonomy'* of these technological developments vis-à-vis other social dynamics. The information technology revolution indeed, Castells comments, was 'instrumental in allowing the implementation of a fundamental process of restructuring of the capitalist system from the 1980s onward' (Castells 2000a: 13). In the process, this technological revolution was 'itself shaped, in its development and manifestations, by the logic and interests of advanced capitalism, *without being reducible to the expression of such interests*' (Castells 2000a: 13, my emphasis). Second, in keeping with his more general move away from any vestige of structural Marxism, Castells places increasing emphasis in his work over time on the *diffusion* or *pervasive effects* of technology within society rather than simply its *economic* significance. It is this latter transition, as Stalder (2006: 27–28) astutely notes, that enables Castells to 'quietly abandon' his concepts of the informational mode of development in favour of the more general concept of '*informationalism*', which can be applied to all domains of society.

Politics: power, experience, identity

Power, for Castells, is 'a *relational* capacity that enables a social actor to influence *asymmetrically* the decisions of other social actors in ways that favour the empowered actors' will, interests and values' (Castells 2009: 10). This in turn, he continues, is exercised in two main ways: (i) by means of '*coercion* (or the possibility of it); and/ or (ii) by the *construction of meaning* as the basis of the discourse through which social actors guide their action', with 'complementary' or 'reciprocal support' between these two main mechanisms of power formation (i.e. coercion–violence; meaning– discourse) (Castells 2009: 10–11).

Clearly then power, as this suggests, 'is more than communication and communication is more than power'. Power nonetheless, Castells stresses:

> ... relies on the control of communication, as counterpower depends on the breaking of such control. And mass communication, the communication that potentially reaches society at large, is shaped and managed by power relationships, rooted in the business of media and the politics of the state.
>
> (Castells 2009: 3)

Communication power therefore, Castells (2009: 3) boldly asserts, 'is at the heart of the structure and dynamics of society' today in the information age.

Related sociological questions also arise, at precisely this juncture, regarding Castells' use of the term 'experience', which is not quite what it may first appear. Take the second book in Castells' information age trilogy for example, *The Power of Identity*. Although, at first glance, this might sound like or suggest a concern with issues of individual minds and meanings, Castells' prime interest here, in keeping with his aforementioned epistemological and methodological stance, is on *groups* and *structures*. Experience therefore is defined in more *collective, empirically observable* terms.

This in turn brings new social movements into sharp focus in Castells' work – defined as 'purposive collective actions whose outcomes, in victory as in defeat, transform the values and institutions of society' (Castells 2010a: 3) – tied as they are to questions of power, politics and identity today. Three ideal types of identity are delineated here in this respect, with new social movements very much aligned or mobilised around the second and third of these. First, *legitimising identity*, 'introduced by the dominant institutions of society to extend and rationalise their domination' (Castells 2010a: 8), thereby resulting, by and large, in the reproduction of the status quo. Second, *resistance identity*, 'generated by those actors who are in positions/conditions devalued and/or stigmatized by the logic of domination, thus building trenches of resistance and survival on the basis of principles different from, or opposed to, those permeating the institutions of society' (Castells 2010a: 8). The emphasis, in this regard, is not so much one of integration as separation and the promotion of challenge and change from *outside* the dominant institutions or values of society. Castells, for example, talks here of the 'exclusion of the excluders by the excluded' as in cases, say, of indigenous movements, fundamentalisms of various kinds, extreme nationalist movements, cults and so on. Finally, *project identity*, for Castells, denotes a situation whereby 'social actors ... build a new identity that redefines their position in society and, by so doing, seek the transformation of overall social structure' (Castells 2010a: 8). The aim here, we might say, is not simply one of integration, but of *integration through transformation* of dominant social institutions and values, as in the case of feminism (vis-à-vis patriarchy) and environmentalism, based on a revaluation of our relationship to nature and ecosphere.

The state too, Castells stresses, is undergoing a more or less profound transformation today in the information age and the network society. It is no longer indeed simply a question of the nation-state, he suggests, but of the *'network state'*, conceived as a system of governance involving *flexible* collaboration and competition between various state and non-state actors. Politics, moreover, expanding on these foregoing themes, becomes primarily *'informational politics'* in the information age; a politics, that is to say, closely associated with the decline of political parties and the increasingly important role of the (new) media system. Not all politics are media politics of course, Castells notes. 'All parties' nonetheless, he argues, 'must go through the media to affect decision-making'. Thus, *'politics is fundamentally framed in its substance, organisation, processes and leadership, by the inherent logic of the media system, particularly the new electronic media'* (Castells 2009: 375): hence the notion of *communication power* as the fundamental form of power in the information age.

A final important sociological aspect of Castells' theory of power, politics, identity and experience bears further comment here, namely, that it is no longer so much a question of domination or repression as *exclusion* that characterises the operation of power and politics today in the information age. Large sectors of the world population, in other words, are effectively bypassed, excluded, marginalised or otherwise rendered 'redundant' in and through these global flows of power and wealth tied to the dominance of informational capitalism and the associated rise of flexible networks. It is in this sense that Castells refers to the multiple 'black holes' of informational capitalism – from the many deprived and excluded black neighbourhoods of America to vast regions of Africa – which he defines collectively as the *'fourth world'*.

Organisation: networks, nodes and the space of flows

Reference has already been made to the notion of networks that, alongside information flows, constitute key components of Castells' analysis of contemporary society and social change.

So what then is a network for Castells and what does he mean by the space of flows? Surprisingly perhaps, given the centrality of the concept within his work, Castells devotes precious little time or space to defining networks in anything other than the most abstract, formal and general of terms. 'A network', he tells us, 'is a set of interconnected nodes. A node is the point at which a network intersects itself' (Castells 2000a: 501). Viewed in the light of Castells' epistemological and methodological stance, however, this is perfectly in keeping with his flexible approach to theory and concepts: a strategy perfectly suited, that is to say, to accommodating a wide range of empirical examples or case studies.

Let us leave aside for a moment the merits or otherwise of this formal sociological definition of networks and its relations, or lack of them to be more precise, to other relevant work in network studies today. Instead let us turn to the pertinent sociological question of whether, and if so why, networks are the predominant form of social organisation today. Networks, after all, are hardly new in the history of humanity or modernity. So what is so novel or distinctive about them today for Castells? Why networks *now* in short? Castells, on this count, is unequivocal. Yes, networks have of course existed in some shape, sense, or form in past epochs or eras, he readily concedes, but not as the *predominant* form of social organisation and certainly not in their current *technologically facilitated, information driven, form*. The reason for the predominance of networks today, in other words, is fundamentally technological. Networks are *complex forms of organisation*, characterised by *flexibility*, 'de-centralising capacity' and 'variable geometry', courtesy of new information and communication technologies, which in turn give rise to new communication-rich environments for action. Networks in this sense, Castells insists, are *always information networks*, involving heterogeneous social actors, coordinated through electronic information flows, but characterised by a high degree of organisational flexibility.

Stalder (2006) casts further helpful light on these matters. A network, he states:

> ... is an enduring pattern of interaction among heterogeneous actors that define one another (identity). They coordinate themselves on the basis of common protocols, values and goals (process). A network reacts nondeterministically to self-selected external influences, thus not simply representing the environment but actively creating it (interdependence). Key properties of a network are emergent from these processes unfolding over time, rather than determined by any of its elements.
>
> (Stalder 2006: 180)

Defined in these terms, Castells' work therefore shares considerable ground here, as Stalder (2006: 183–84) notes, with recent developments in 'complexity theory' and the new 'science of networks'. [2, 3] That it takes commentators like Stalder, however, to elucidate these links and spell these formal properties of networks out is itself nonetheless, to repeat, characteristic or symptomatic of Castells' own somewhat different concerns and preoccupations.

The key points for our purposes nonetheless, these links and connections notwithstanding, are as follows: (i) networks, for Castells, are not simply new *enduring* forms of organisation but the *primary* or *predominant* forms of social organisation today through a pervasive '*network logic*' that permeates all domains of life; (ii) informationalism and networking are intimately yet *contingently* connected in *complex, dynamic, reciprocal, mutually reinforcing* if not non-linear ways – informationalism being a technological matter, networking a question of social morphology (Stalder 2006: 186) – in the new age or era of *informational capitalism*.

These developments in informationalism and networking are in turn implicated in further transformations of time and space today. Here we encounter another of Castells' key concepts, namely the *space of flows*. Space and time, he notes, are 'fundamental material dimensions of human life' (Castells 2000a: 407). To the extent however that contemporary society is organised around flows – of information, technology, organisational interaction, images, sounds, symbols, and so forth – and to the extent that these flows are not just one dimension or element of social organisation but prime expressions of processes that have now come to dominate our economic, political and symbolic life – then it is indeed timely and legitimate to refer to the 'space of flows' as the '*material organization of time-sharing practices that work through flows*' (Castells 2000a: 442). The space of flows, in other words, is intended to convey the ever-increasing role these new electronic circuits and continuous flows of communication – *at a distance* yet in *simultaneous time* – are coming to play in the information age and the network society.

Castells further specifies this rather abstract concept in terms of three material levels or layers of support, which taken together, he suggests, 'constitute the space of flows'. First, a '*circuit of electronic exchanges*' (e.g. micro-electronics-based, telecommunications, computer processing, broadcasting systems and so on); second, the '*nodes and hubs*' that make up informational networks; and third, the '*spatial organisation of the dominant managerial elites* (rather than classes, of which more later) that exercise the directional functions around which such space is articulated' (Castells 2000a: 442–45).

The space of flows, however, is perhaps best understood in terms of its opposite, namely the *historically rooted* spatial organisation of our common *embodied experience*, which Castells terms the *space of places*. The space of flows, he notes, does 'not penetrate down to the whole realm of human experience in the network society'. The 'overwhelming majority of people', indeed Castells stresses, in advanced and traditional societies alike, 'live in places and so they perceive their space as placebased' (Castells 2000a: 453). Viewed in this light then, it is perhaps not too much of an oversimplification to think of the space of flows as a kind of 'placeless space', 'power', and 'logic' vis-à-vis the 'space of places'; the two conceived in dynamic terms to one another, which, Castells stresses, are 'not predetermined in their outcome'. Thus people do still live in places of course, but:

> ... because function and power in our societies are organized in the space of flows, the structural domination of its logic essentially alters the meaning and dynamics of places. Experience, by being related to places, becomes abstracted from power and meaning is increasingly separated from knowledge. There follows a *structural schizophrenia* between two spatial logics that threatens to break down communication channels in society. The *dominant tendency is toward a horizon of networked, ahistorical space of flows, aiming at imposing its logic over scattered, segmented places, increasingly unrelated to each other, less and less able to share cultural codes.*
>
> (Castells 2000a: 458–59; my emphasis)

Space and time, flows and places, globalisation and localisation, inclusion and exclusion, these then constitute key dimensions and dynamics of power and politics for Castells in the network society and the information age. Unless 'cultural, political and physical bridges are built between these two forms of space', moreover, Castells warns, 'we may be heading toward life in parallel universes whose times cannot meet because they are warped into different dimensions of a social hyperspace' (2000a: 459).

A 'neuro' turn? Brains, minds and meanings

> The most fundamental form of power lies in its ability to shape the human mind.
>
> (Castells 2009: 3, my emphasis)

A notable shift in Castells' more recent work – given his former more collective emphasis on 'experience' and 'identity' in terms of groups, structures, and empirically observable phenomena, and his general methodological commitment to social morphology over action – is his willingness to engage not simply with minds and meanings, but brains and neural networks.

On the one hand then, this is not simply a notable but a significant or seismic shift of focus, which straddles both different levels of analysis and different disciplines. On the other hand, however, it underlines once again Castells' aforementioned pragmatic stance toward theoretical matters. For someone interested in networks of any kind, moreover, then neural networks are perhaps fair game too. To neglect them indeed may well be a significant omission, particularly when it is communication power in the information age you are interested in.

Others in the social sciences and humanities today are of a similar mindset. Whilst Castells indeed, in characteristic fashion, has little or no interest in positioning his work within past or present sociological traditions of theory, his latest work on *Communication Power* (2009) can nonetheless be read as part and parcel of something approaching a 'neuro' turn in the social sciences and humanities, including new hybrid fields of inquiry such as neuroeconomics, neuropolitics, neurohistory, neuroaesthetics, even neurosociology, neuropsychonanalysis, and neurotheology.

Castells' own particular interests in this regard, in keeping with some of these hybrid fields of inquiry, is less on the social shaping of neuroscience than the ways in which findings from neuroscience can be drawn upon in order to *deepen* and *enrich* his own analysis of communication power in the information age and the network society. Viewed in this light indeed, it may not be too fanciful to suggest that Castells' analysis here constitutes a prime example of a neurosociology or a neuropolitics in the information age, even if he himself might quibble with any such moniker.

If we are to fully understand the construction of *power* relationships through *communication* in the global network society, Castells now argues, we need to appreciate that this is not simply a matter of structural determinants, but of cognitive processing through minds and meanings. 'If power works by acting on the human mind by means of communicating messages', that is to say, 'we need to understand how the human mind processes these messages, and how this processing translates into the political realm' (Castells 2009: 6–7).

Castells' prime sources here – taking the systematic campaign of misinforming the American public by the Bush administration over the Iraq war as his case study – derive from recent findings in fields such as affective intelligence, political communication, and political psychology, which themselves draw upon new research in neuroscience and cognitive science, particularly the work of Damasio (2003, 2000, 1994).[4] These sources, Castells suggests, provide a 'most-needed bridge between social structuration and the individual processing of power relationships' (Castells 2009: 7).

Turning now to the Iraq war drama, the key issue here for Castells, it seems, turns on the implantation into the minds of millions of people of two extremely powerful 'frames' of reference, pertaining respectively to the 'war on terror' and 'patriotism'. The war on terror and its associated themes and images, for example:

> ... constructed a *network of associations in people's minds* ... They *activated the deepest emotion in the human brain*: the *fear* of death. Psychological experiments in a plurality of contexts provide evidence that connecting issues and events with death *favours conservative political attitudes in people's brains*.
>
> (Castells 2009: 169)

These processes, as this suggests, are largely *affective* or *emotional* rather than simply *rational*, with politicians skilled in how to solicit proper emotions and win not simply the minds but the hearts of people; the upshot being that the 'rational analysis of power-making processes starts with a recognition of the *limits* of rationality in the process'.[5] The way 'we feel', in short, structures 'the way we think, and ultimately the way we act' (Castells 2009: 192).

Appraising Castells: a balance sheet

Hints of an appraisal of Castells' work are already evident in the discussion. It is high time nonetheless that we addressed these matters foursquare, albeit briefly given the constraints of space, through a succinct balance sheet of sorts.

A number of points are worth stressing in this respect, with the interested reader directed, once again, to the authoritative, informative, and extensive accounts and appraisals of Castells' work noted previously – see for example Van Dijk (1999); Calhoun (2000a); Jessop (2003); Webster (2002); Webster and Dimitriou (2004).

First and foremost, on the positive side of the balance sheet, despite his own somewhat pragmatic stance towards theoretical matters, Castells is undoubtedly a major sociological theorist of our times, providing as he does a more or less coherent if not complete or comprehensive account of the network society and the information age. This is no small achievement. It has also garnered favourable comparisons, in terms of scope, substance and style, with the sociological classics, notably Marx and Weber. Giddens, for example, in his review of the network society in the *Times Higher Education Supplement*, puts the matter well when he states:

> We live today in a period of intense and puzzling transformation, signalling perhaps a move beyond the industrial era altogether. Yet where are the great sociological works that chart this transformation? Hence the importance of Manuel Castells' multivolume work, in which he seeks to chart the social and economic dynamics of the information age. It would not be fanciful to compare the work to Max Weber's *Economy and Society*, written almost a century earlier ... [It] is bound to be a major reference source for years to come.
> (Giddens 1996: e-version)

Castells' analyses of informational capitalism, informationalism, the space of flows, the space of places, network logic, communication power, real virtuality, together with detailed case studies of new social movements and rise of fundamentalisms (both Christian and Muslim), are certainly major accomplishments. So too is his more recent attempt to deepen or enrich this work through links to modern-day neuroscience, albeit in ways to repeat that largely emphasise the social import rather than the social shaping of the latter.[6]

A number of tensions or problems nonetheless may be pointed to here in Castells' work; some of which remain valid to the present day, others partly addressed or overcome in his more recent writings.

The first of these returns us to the question of '*determinism*' touched on earlier. Is Castells, we might ask, vulnerable to the charge of technological determinism; a case, in other words, of putting technology very firmly in the driving seat of social transformation and change in the information age? The answer it seems, as Castells himself admits, is a qualified 'yes and no', which for our purposes equates to something like a '*soft*' or '*weak*' determinism. Consider, for example, Castells' rejoinder to Calhoun, Lyon and Touraine in *Prometheus*, in which he asks and answers this very question as to whether or not this amounts to 'technological determinism':

> Yes and no. Fundamentally no, because I do not say (and no one in their right mind would say) that technology determines society ... But yes, if you want, in a particular sense, without new technologies, there could be no economic globalisation, no network enterprise, no global media, no global communication, and no global criminal economy.
>
> (Castells 2000b: 137)

A related cluster of issues here concern what Stalder (2006: 196) terms the 'pre-eminence of morphology over action' in Castells' work, thereby resulting in various charges of 'reifying networks'; of not giving due attention to the *mutual* shaping of structure and action; of conjuring up a 'one dimensional' network society, and so forth – see, for example, van Dijk (1999) and Marcuse (2002) on these counts. These to be sure are important criticisms. These charges nonetheless are partly addressed in Castells' more recent work, such as *Communication Power* (2009), in which greater attention is placed on the *struggle* over networks and forms of *counterpower*, including the programming and reprogramming of networks.

Another notable if not significant sociological omission, particularly for someone with (former) Marxist credentials, is any notion of a *capitalist or global class*, which therefore leaves Castells open to the charge of focusing more on the *excluded* than the *excluders* (Marcuse 2002). To think or speak in such terms nonetheless, for Castells, would be to mistakenly attribute agency and control to a 'class' or group who themselves are caught up, and hence subject to, the 'mighty whirlwind' of faceless capitalism and the uncertainties of global financial markets: a complex, constantly changing configuration or reconfiguration of power and networks, that is to say. Conflict moreover is no longer primarily articulated around questions and issues to do with who owns the means of production. Castells then in this regard, as Stalder (2006: 191) comments, appears more comfortable speaking of a 'global elite' than a capitalist or global class, with a focus on a 'shared culture' facilitated through communication in the global networks of power and wealth.

It is also somewhat curious, as Stalder (2006: 204) rightly notes, that a theorist of the information age neglects or omits what is perhaps a key if not defining new commodity form in the information age, namely *intellectual property* in the shape of copyright, patents, trademarks; commodity forms that now include or extend, of course, to the very technologies of life that Castells all too briefly discusses, in the guise of important new forms of biovalue, bioprospecting and biopatenting in the bioeconomy (cf. Rose 2007; Fuller 2006).

Fuller (1999) also draws attention to another significant omission in Castells' work, namely the role of the academy in the information age. This includes a notable absence of any significant degree of reflexivity about the material conditions of production of Castells' own data sources and intellectual outputs in his elite information-rich sector of the academy. For someone who places great emphasis on empirical data collection, moreover, Fuller comments, the limits of his own data sources are significantly underplayed, not least with regard to his claims about the decline or demise of the nation-state. If the 'network society', in other words:

... is indeed the 'space of flows' bounded by global financial markets and pockets of local resistance, both of which are in their own way 'privatised', the publicly available statistics compiled by the United Nations, the European Union, the International Monetary Fund and the World Bank are prima facie little more than the effects of hypothetical processes for which Castells provides no direct statistical demonstration.

(Fuller 1999: 164–65)

If we add to this Castells' indifference, by and large, to connecting, placing, or situating his writings in relation to other relevant bodies of thought and research, both past and present, then this perhaps suggests a mixed bag of pros and cons as to the merits of his work and its links and legacies for the future.

Again, however, we return full circle here to the first point above, namely that Castells' theory of the network society and information age is still nonetheless a major sociological accomplishment, and a rich resource to mine, extend and develop in contemporary sociology and beyond. It is to these very matters, therefore, with health in mind so to speak, that we now turn in the next section of the chapter.

Applications: sleep and health in the network society

Doubtless there are many 'applications' we could make in order to illustrate the relevance of Castells' work to health, medicine, and society. Some of these Castells provides himself, such as his, albeit brief and selective, engagements with developments in biotechnology (or 'technologies of life' as he nicely terms them), and his analysis of 'death denied' in the network society. We might also, of course, profitably apply Castells' analysis of new social movements to the health domain, given growing interests in social movements and health in recent years (see for example Brown and Zavestoki 2005).

In what follows, however, I take a somewhat different or novel line, which at first glance may seem far removed not simply from Castells' central sociological concerns and preoccupations, but from sociology in general, health related or otherwise. I am talking about recent sociological interest in sleep, health, and society, including my own contributions to this rich new vein of sociological research over the past decade or so (see for example Williams 2011; 2005; 2002; Williams and Bendelow 1998).

How then, if at all, is Castells relevant here? Or to put it slightly differently, can profitable relays be forged back and forth between Castells' analysis of the network society in the information age and recent sociological engagements with sleep, health, and society?

The answer I venture, unsurprisingly perhaps, is a provisional yes on at least three main counts.

The protesting body? Sleep, timeless time, and social arrhythmia

Our starting point here concerns the alleged 'problem' of sleep today in contemporary society. Sleep it is claimed is fast becoming a casualty of contemporary life and living in the incandescent if not incessant, around-the-clock, 24/7 age or era, the cost and consequence of which have yet to be fully counted.

Dement, for example, a leading US sleep expert, claims that: (i) we are a 'sleep sick society'; (ii) people now sleep on average one and a half hours less each night than they would have a century ago; (iii) there is an 'epidemic' of sleep deprivation today; and that (iv) most people in advanced industrialised countries are walking around with an accumulated 'sleep deficit' of between 25–30 hours. A litany of supposedly sleepy people are pointed to in this regard, by sleep experts, commentators, and critics alike – from sleepy drivers to sleepy doctors, sleepy pilots to sleepy parents, not to mention sleepy politicians – thereby underlining not simply the extent of the problem today but the significant risks short sleep or poor sleep poses for public health and safety.

Many of these discourses and debates are American in origin. Attention to sleep matters nonetheless is increasingly evident elsewhere too. A recent report by the Mental Health Foundation (2011) for example – based on findings from the Great British Sleep Survey – suggests that up to a third of the population may suffer from insomnia, with important implications for mental and physical health. Early findings from the large-scale ESRC *Understanding Society* project[7] also indicated that 12 per cent of respondents report very short sleep of under six hours per night, with an additional 16 per cent reporting sleep of under six and a half hours. Women moreover, the survey finds, are consistently more likely than men to have self-reported sleep problems (Arber and Meadows 2011).

It is not my intention to rehearse the finer details of these data and debates again here – see Williams (2011, 2005) for example for extensive discussions of these sleep matters. Suffice it to say, for present purposes, that recourse to Castells adds further potentially useful sociological dimensions to these debates, particularly in terms of the drivers and dynamics of these sleep problems today.

Castells' analysis of the space of flows in terms of time–space relations, for example, is potentially useful here, casting further critical sociological light on the increasingly fraught, problematic or vexed relationship between sleep, technology and time today in the information age. Part and parcel of a wide range of debates on the compression or reconfiguration of time–space in late or post-modernity; the blurring or erasure of boundaries such as home and work, the public and the private; and the 'acceleration of just about everything' these days through the 'dictatorship of speed' in this supposedly 'go-faster' phase of global capitalism (cf. Harvey 1989, Giddens 1991, Virilio 1986/1977; Gleick 2000; Agger 2004; Tomlinson 2007). Castells speaks here of our increasingly complex if not chaotic relationship to time in the information age, which amounts not simply to the mixing up and multiplicity of context-dependent temporalities or timeframes, but the advent or emergence of a new temporal regime, namely, '*timeless time*' or 'time-denying-time'.

Timeless time, as this suggests, is paradoxical in that it implies a form of time that is not time so to speak, or not time as we have known it before: a kind of 'post-time', as Stalder (2006: 157) puts it, characterised by the *absence of any fixed sequence* as in say the cyclical time of the medieval period or the mechanical clock time of the industrial era. The 'relentless effort to compress time in all domains of human activity', Castells argues, compressing time 'to the limit' in effect, is 'tantamount to making time sequence, and thus time, disappear' (Castells 2000a: 464). We are moreover, he suggests, witnessing the '*breaking down of the rhythms, either biological or social, associated with the notion of a life-cycle*' (Castells 2000a: 480): a process Castells refers to as a drift towards *social arrhythmia* that, to all intents and purposes, may be regarded as 'another form of the annihilation of time, of human biological time, of the time rhythm by which our species has been regulated since its origins' (Castells 2000a: 480).

These terms, to be sure, are far from problematic: the most speculative parts of Castells' work to date perhaps. They do nonetheless, as Stalder rightly notes, speak to the fact that:

> ... in an increasing number of social processes the rhythms of the clock or those of nature are *no longer dominant* or that they can at least be *substantially distorted*. They *don't disappear completely* as points of reference, but they *interact with a different temporal patterning* based on advanced computing and biological technologies [of life]. *Established sequences* of when things are done, throughout the day, and throughout a person's life, are being *mixed up* for a growing number of people.
>
> (Stalder 2006: 160 my emphasis)

Thinking these issues through with sleep in mind, I venture, is instructive on a number of counts. It does not indeed involve too great a stretch or leap of the sociological imagination to claim that sleep, like waking life, is closely bound up with these dynamics of timeless time and social arrhythmia today in the network society and information age. The more these trends towards timeless time accelerate in the information age for example, and the more disturbed or disordered, perturbed or problematic, severed or subordinated our connections to the cyclical or biological rhythms of life become through the associated drift towards social arrhythmia, the more sleep problems escalate or multiply.

Sleep in this regard, we might say, expresses and embodies not simply the *dynamics* but the *dilemmas* of timeless time and social arrhythmia in the information age today. Why? Well precisely because, for better or worse, the sleep–wake cycle remains stubbornly attuned or geared towards these age-old biological, or chronobiological, rhythms of life. We may all, in other words, trade or toil under the escalating demands and dictates if not the tyrannies of these new temporal or timeless regimes, we may even come to regard tiredness or sleepiness as a 'normal' part of modern day life and living (Widerberg 2006), but our bodies clearly do so under protest: hence the problems of shift work, jet lag, and the more widespread problems of sleep deprivation or sleepiness in these restless if not relentless times or timeless times of ours.

From here indeed it is but a short step to a further, perhaps more radical, sociological interpretation of sleep that itself casts further critical light, if not doubt, on Castells' very notion of timeless time. Sleep, that is to say, not simply as a powerful corporeal reminder of these biological rhythms of life and the limits of our conscious waking involvements in society, but a powerful or potent site and source of corporeal *conflict, protest, refusal* or *resistance* in the 24/7 society and the wired-awake world: a chronobiological critique, in effect, of this supposedly new form of timeless time and social arrhythmia in the information age.

Castells it seems may agree, or not entirely disagree at least. 'People and societies', he notes, ignore the biological rhythms of life 'at their peril' (Castells 2000a: 475). To the extent moreover, to repeat, that timeless time is not really about the absence of time at all but about our increasingly complex if not chaotic relationship to mixed and multiple temporalities that clash, compete, or cancel one another out, then sleep again fits more or less readily into the picture here as a novel yet vital example.

Whatever our interpretation of these matters however, the broader sociological point surely remains, namely that many of our sleep problems today, recalling Mills' (1959) '*Sociological Imagination*', provide another prime example of the link between personal troubles and public issues, albeit in times very different today to those envisaged by Mills over half a century ago now.

Rethinking medicalisation? Sleep and health in the information age

A second obvious connection or nexus here concerns the potentially powerful role that information and communication technologies (ICTs) now play, not simply in potentially or problematically reconfiguring our sleep 'time' in the wired world, but in the very construction, monitoring, and management of sleep as a vital matter today both inside and outside the laboratory or clinic.

Castells' work in this regard resonates with rich and vibrant new streams of sociological work over the past decade or so on the media, medicine, and health – including traditional broadcasting and print news media (Seale 2003) and new media such as the internet (Hardy 2001; Nettleton *et al.* 2005; Miah and Rich 2007), as well as related work on the social dimensions and dynamics of so-called e-health technologies and virtual medicine (Waldby 2000) – connections albeit that these authors by and large fail to make given the general neglect of Castells' work within medical sociology to date, information-related or otherwise.

The sleep laboratory and the sleep clinic of course are obvious reference points here in terms of the use of information-related tools and technologies to monitor, measure, and manage sleep (Williams 2011). It is to three other key examples however, beyond the lab or clinic so to speak, that we now turn, each illustrative I suggest of the dynamic role of various media in sleep matters today, and each ripe for sociological links or relays to Castells' analysis of 'communication power' in the information age and the network society.

First, and still perhaps foremost, broadcasting and print news media continue to play important roles in the construction and framing of sleep matters or sleep problems in popular culture. This for instance, as recent sociological research has shown, includes the role of the media in various forms of 'disease mongering' regarding conditions such as restless legs syndrome (Woloshin and Schwartz 2006;

Moynihan and Cassells 2005), and the differential construction of sleep problems such as snoring and insomnia as more or less medicalised conditions or public health issues (Williams *et al.* 2008; Seale *et al.* 2007). It also, of course, includes shifting media portrayals of biomedical technologies associated with sleep such as sleeping tablets, which have become increasingly critical over time (Gabe and Bury 1996), and ambivalent media constructions of newer drugs, such as the wakefulness-promoting agent Modafinil, particularly for 'enhancement' rather than 'therapeutic' purposes in the 24/7 society amongst the otherwise 'healthy' (Williams *et al.* 2009; Coveney *et al.* 2009).

It is not simply a case of media constructions of sleep, however, but of the role various media are now increasingly coming to play in the very shaping and (self) diagnosis of sleep problems today. Cases or charges of so-called 'disease mongering', for instance, have already been mentioned above. One does not have to resort to any such notions however in order to appreciate the dynamic role of the media, particularly new media, in the configuration of diseases, disorders, and diagnoses today. Type the keywords 'sleepy', 'sleepiness', or 'drowsiness' into any internet search engine for instance, as Kroll-Smith (2003) rightly remarks, and many if not most hits will portray this as some variant of 'excessive daytime sleepiness' (EDS). The impression that this is or may be a distinct disorder, moreover, he notes, is conveyed in a variety of ways, including: (i) omission in discussions of EDS of any obvious or explicit reference to it as a 'symptom'; (ii) the manner in which the very name 'excessive daytime sleepiness' and the acronym EDS imply 'a more significant identity as a bona fide medical disorder'; and (iii) the readily available and multiple websites for *online self-diagnostic tests* such as the Epworth Sleepiness Scale (ESS), which might 'easily assume a somatic reality against which a number becomes a meaningful piece of evidence about the relative presence or absence of a particular disorder' (Kroll-Smith 2003: 637).

Challenges to these expert renditions of sleep matters, effective or otherwise, are also now of course increasingly possible through the internet. Weisgerber's (2004) study of an online forum for sleep paralysis, for example, highlights the way in which dominant scientific understandings and explanations of this terrifying condition are actively resisted or rejected by participants in favour of other powerful spiritual or supernatural explanations based on long-established traditions in folklore.

Our third and perhaps most novel example, however, highlights the role of *mobile* information and communication technologies in the very monitoring and management of our sleep far away from the sleep lab or clinic, in the comfort of our own homes whilst we sleep! A variety of 'apps', for example, are now ready and available to download for use on your mobile phone with sleep in mind. These for instance, in keeping with other long-established technologies such as watch actigraphy or sleeptracker watches, promise to monitor or measure your sleep, tell you if or when you snore, even help you improve your sleep (hygiene) in order to get that elusive yet vital good night's sleep.

Clearly more could be said in terms of each of these foregoing examples. The key point for present purposes, nonetheless, is that each illustrates in their different ways the dynamic configuration or reconfiguration of sleep matters in the information age far away from the sleep lab or the sleep clinic.

This in turn therefore invites further important sociological reflections on the very nature and dynamics of medicalisation today, both sleep specific and in general, in the information age. The argument here, succinctly stated, is that reading or rereading these issues through Castells invites or encourages us to think not simply about a new era of *informational capitalism* but a new phase of *informational medicine* in the network society that *extends far beyond the institutional confines and contexts of medicine in the past, even the recent past*.

Nettleton (2004), for example, drawing on De Mul's (1999) theorisation of the 'informationalization of the world view' usefully speaks here, through a term apparently suggested to her by Webster (2002), of a new phase of 'e-scaped medicine' involving an 'elective affinity' between this new 'medical cosmology' (cf. Jewson 1976) and contemporary socio-technological changes associated with the information and communications technology revolution. This moreover, she emphasises, involves a double point of reference in which medical *knowledge*, transmuted into medical or health-related *information, escapes* its traditional institutional confines through a process of *e-scaping* – the latter enabling extraordinary flows of information through networks and nodes at lightening speeds across compressed time-space. Medical knowledge, in other words, is therefore:

> ... no longer exclusive to the medical academy and the formal medical text. It has 'escaped' into the *networks* of contemporary *information scapes* where it can be accessed and re-appropriated. Rather than being concealed within the institutional domains of medicine, knowledge of the biophysical body has *seeped out* into cyberspace ... As medical knowledge 'escapes' moreover and is 'e-scaped' the ability of the medical professional or laboratory scientist to shape the content of medical knowledge diminishes.
> (Nettleton 2004: 675–76, my emphasis)

Kroll-Smith (2003) too arrives at broadly similar conclusions, albeit with different intellectual debts, in his aforementioned paper on EDS in popular culture. The case of EDS, he suggests:

> ... hints at an evocative idea, to wit, the 'voice of medicine' and the 'voice of the life-world' are beginning to converse *outside the solid containers of institutional medicine*. The 'voice of medicine', it appears, is escaping into a contemporary world of porous institutions increasingly affected and affecting one another in a delightful, if maddening, exchange of digital, video and print media.

The institutional authority of medicine remains a political fact in the day-to-day lives of ordinary people of course, as Kroll-Smith himself acknowledges. Illustrated in his inquiry nonetheless, he insists, is 'an alternative authority expressed in the voice of print and digital media': a case, in short, of locating medical knowledge 'outside of its institutional matrix in *less solidified, more casual and contingent venues*' (Kroll-Smith 2003: 640).

The similarities and resonances here to Castells' work are striking, even if these authors don't make them. Perhaps therefore, in keeping with recent ongoing sociological debates about the shifting engines of medicalisation (Conrad 2007) or biomedicalisation (Clarke et al. 2003),[8] we might profitably refer here not simply to a new phase of informational medicine but of 'e-scaped' or '*i-scaped*' *medicalisation* or biomedicalisation today in the information age and the network society.

Recourse to Castells however, in the grand sociological tradition, also encourages us to go much further here on a number of counts. A full and proper sociological understanding of communication power in the information age for example, he reminds us, requires the integration of three key components of these processes, namely:

the 'structural determinants of social and political power in the global network society';
the 'structural determinants of the process of mass communication under the organizational, cultural and technological conditions of our time'; and
the 'cognitive processing of the signals presented by the communication system to the human mind as it relates to politically relevant social practice'.

(Castells 2000a: 8)

There is no significant gap here moreover, Castells stresses, between the material and symbolic realms of social life. All realities indeed, he notes, are communicated in and through the symbolic. What is 'historically specific' to the new communication system therefore, organised around electronic flows of information, is 'not its inducement of virtual reality, but the construction of *real virtuality*' whereby:

> All messages of all kinds become enclosed in the medium because the medium has become so comprehensive, so diversified, so malleable, that it absorbs in the same multimedia text the whole of human experience, past, present, and future.
>
> (Castells 2000a: 403–04)

Finally, as a flag for future sociological research in medical sociology as elsewhere no doubt, Castells points to another key form of communication power today in the guise of what he terms '*mass self-communication*'; a new communication system, built through messaging, social networking sites, and blogging, which is already, he claims, having profound implications for power relationships in the network society.

Networked sleep? The sleep industry and beyond

Our last application or illustration, in this chapter at least, returns us to the very question of networks and their relevance or otherwise to sleep. We might usefully pose the matter here in the following provocative terms: what on earth has sleep, surely the most personal or private if not asocial of things, got to do with 'networks' let alone the 'network society'?

In part, of course, we have already answered this in the foregoing discussion. Other important sociological dimensions to the picture, however, also come into view here by turning foursquare to the very question of sleep-related networks of various kinds.

Sleep it turns out, like all other aspects of our lives these days, is indeed networked in all sorts of ways, some more surprising than others (Crossley 2004; Williams and Crossley 2008).[9] *When* I sleep, *how* I sleep, *where* I sleep, not to mention with *whom* I sleep and *what* meanings and values we accord sleep, are all, for starters, shaped or influenced by the networks we live in, work in, and sleep in, both day and night. Sleep in other words is never an entirely private or personal matter and the sleeper is never an entirely individual or isolated sleeper. The construction and configuration, monitoring and management of sleep is also, of course, as we have seen, in no small part a product of the multiple communication networks and information flows evident today in the network society.

Perhaps most obviously however, we may point to the 'sleep industry' as a multiply networked and rapidly expanding or escalating enterprise. This for example includes both the 'commercial' and the 'therapeutic' wings of the sleep industry; distinctions that themselves of course are far from clear cut or watertight given significant elements of overlap between the commercial and the therapeutic wings, particularly in the US.

The commercial wing, for instance, includes everything from the bed and mattress industry and associated sales of bedding and nightwear, to companies such as Metro Naps who specialise in the provision of napping pods – not to mention sleep-themed hotels, from the economy to the luxury end of the market, who promise their guest a sound or perfect night's slumber.

The therapeutic wing, in contrast, spans everything from sleep laboratories, sleep clinics (a fast-growing sector in North America today) and the associated diagnostics, drugs, and devices markets, to over-the-counter sleep aids, alternative remedies and a booming self-help industry of books, CDs, and DVDs of the 'how-to' kind – i.e. how to get a 'good' night's sleep, how to 'improve' your sleep in one way or another in the name of health, happiness, productivity, performance, wisdom, virtue, and so forth. This moreover, as we previously noted, now even includes downloadable sleep-related apps for your mobile phone, which again serve to further blur the commercial/therapeutic distinction drawn above.

To this of course we may add a variety of other advocacy, patient, and pressure groups or organisations, such as the National Sleep Foundation (NSF) in North America – a networked organisation *par excellence* with the official motto 'Alerting the public, healthcare providers and policymakers to the life-and-death importance of adequate sleep' (www.sleepfoundation.org) – which directly or indirectly are busy campaigning on various sleep-related fronts.

Again a detailed tracing or mapping of these issues in networked terms is alas beyond the scope of the present chapter. Suffice it to say that networks of various kinds are clearly involved here. Further analysis along these lines therefore, I suggest, would not simply add valuable new dimensions to sociological work on sleep, health, and society to date, but provide another important relay back and forth to Castells' work, as well as many other writers and researchers today who are now increasingly turning their attention to 'networks' of various kinds, health-related or otherwise – see for example Christakis and Fowler (2009).

Concluding remarks

Let me end with a few brief concluding remarks on the relevance, or otherwise, of Castells' work at a time of what might best be described as one of sociological *renewal* (cf. Osborne and Rose 2008). If sociology indeed is currently in the process of discussing and debating its own complexities if not challenges or crises (cf. McLennan 2003; Urry 2003; Fuller 2006; Savage and Burrows 2007), and reflexively constructing or lamenting its own futures, then where exactly does Castells' work fit or sit within all this fermentation and flux?

On the one hand of course, recalling Giddens' appraisal once more, the answer to this question is fairly simple and straightforward. Castells' work remains a major reference source on the social and economic dynamics of the information age, and our place within it, justifiably earning him favourable comparisons to other works in the great or grand sociological tradition, and accolades such as the C. Wright Mills Award. To the extent moreover that Castells' writings resonate with wider contemporary sociological debates to do with global complexity, networks, flows, mobilities, and the like (cf. Urry 2003; 2000), then he is indeed a key resource or vital ingredient in any such sociological 'renewal'. Part and parcel, that is to say, of a sociology 'on the move', to invoke the title of the recent XVII World Congress of Sociology, which in the words of the ISA president Michel Wieviorka involves 'new objects of research', 'new approaches', the re-evaluation of sociology's own 'rich heritage', and a 'new openness with regard to other disciplines and to normative questions' – all of which, Wieviorka stresses, are essential to the continuing 'vitality of our discipline' (http://www.isa-sociology.org/congress2010/, accessed 14 April 2011).

On the other hand, however, Castells' own reluctance to situate or connect his work in terms of these wider developments and debates in sociology, complexity theory, network studies, and the like, coupled with his largely 'pragmatic' or 'tool box' approach to theory, means that he is not perhaps as widely read or extensively referenced today, in sociology at least, as he might otherwise be: an 'eclipsing' of an early trail blazer maybe as these wider developments and debates take off in sociology and cognate fields?

Here too of course we return full circle to the neglect of Castells' work within medical sociology to date, which this chapter in its own small way has sought to rectify. There are certainly, I have suggested, plenty of rich relays here for medical sociologists to mine and explore in years to come, as my own particular case study of the sleep, health, and society nexus exemplifies. Future research on health and social movements, moreover, would doubtless find much of value to think both with and against in Castells' work on the power and politics of identity in the information age.

Castells then, to conclude, certainly repays close reading, or rereading, in this light. To the extent moreover that this chapter achieves its aim and stimulates further interest in Castells' work within medical sociology, it will be interesting to see how these connections are taken up and developed in years to come: another rich resource in medical sociology's own *renewal* in the twenty-first century and the information age perhaps. Watch this space ...

Notes

1 Soviet statism failed in its attempts at restructuring, in Castells' view, in large part because of its 'incapacity ... to assimilate and use the principles of informationalism embodied in the new information technologies' (2000a: 13). Chinese statism in contrast seemed to succeed 'by shifting from statism to state-led capitalism and integration in global economic networks' (Castells 2000a: 13) – see volume III (Castells 2010b) of the information trilogy for a discussion of both cases.
2 See Gleick (1987) and Urry (2003), for example, on chaos and global complexity.
3 Castells indeed, Stalder (2006: 170) notes, is not only 'extremely frugal' in his definition of networks, he also does not use or even refer to any standard categories of metrics (e.g. density of connections, number of links, symmetry of communication) developed by network analysts. See, for example, Chistakis and Fowler (2009); Watts (2003); Monge and Contractor (2003); Barabási (2002); Wasserman and Faust (1994).
4 Damasio indeed provides the following ringing endorsement of the book on the back: *'Manuel Castells unites the mind of a social scientist with the soul of an artist. His trilogy took us to the edge of the millennium. This book takes us beyond the critical crossroads of the 21st century where technology and communication power converge'* (original emphasis).
5 This may at first glance appear strange, given Castells' indebtedness to Damasio's (1994) emphasis on the supportive role emotions play in rational decision making. Reason and emotion nonetheless are still clearly different things for Damasio. Whilst emotion may support rationality, Damasio stresses, it may also sabotage or overthrow it.
6 Science and technology studies (STS), for example, provide rich resources here in terms of the social shaping of science and technology. See for example Hackett *et al.* (2007).
7 A national study tracking 100,000 people in 40,000 British households.
8 Whilst Conrad (2005) refers to the 'shifting engines of medicalisation' and hence retains the concept of medicalisation, Clarke and colleagues (2003) proposed instead the term biomedicalisation given the increasingly techno-social, multi-sited and multi-dimensional character of these processes today.
9 Thanks to Nick Crossley for various discussion along these lines over the years.

References

Agger, B. (2004) *Speeding Up Fast Capitalism: Cultures, Jobs, Families, Schools, Bodies*. Boulder, CO: Paradigm Publishers.
Arber, S. and Meadows, R. (2011) Social and health patterning of sleep quality and duration, in *Understanding Society: Early Findings from the First Wave of the UK's Household Longitudinal Study (Wave 1, Year 1)*. Available at: http://research.understandingsociety.org.uk/findings/early-findings (accessed 31 March 2011).
Barabási, A.-L. (2002) *Linked: The New Science of Networks*. Cambridge, MA: Perseus Books.
Brown, P. and Zavestoki, S. (eds.) (2005) *Social Movements in Health*. Oxford: Blackwell.
Calhoun, C. (2000a) Resisting globalization or shaping it? *Prometheus*. 3: 29–67.

Castells, M. (2010a) *The Information Age: Economy, Society and Culture Volume II: The Power of Identity*, second edition. Oxford: Blackwell.
——(2010b) *The Information Age: Economy, Society and Culture Volume III: End of the Millennium*, second edition. Oxford: Blackwell.
——(2009) *Communication Power*. Oxford: Oxford University Press.
——(2001) *The Internet Galaxy: Reflections on the Internet, Business and Society*. Oxford: Oxford University Press.
——(2000a) *The Information Age: Economy, Society and Culture Volume I: Rise of the Network Society*, second edition. Oxford: Blackwell.
——(2000b) Globalization and identity: a rejoinder to Calhoun, Lyon and Tourain. *Prometheus*. 4: 108–23.
——(1989) *The Informational City: Information Technology, Economic Restructuring and the Urban-Regional Process*. Oxford: Blackwell.
——(1978) *City, Class and Power*. London: Macmillan.
——(1977) *The Urban Question: a Marxist Approach* (transl. A. Sheridan). London: Edward Arnold.
Christakis, N. A. and Fowler, J. H. (2009) *Connected; The Surprising Power of Our Social Networks and How They Shape Our Lives*. New York: Little Brown and Company.
Clarke, A., Mamo, L., Fishman, J. R., Shim, J. K. and Fosket, J. R. (2003) Biomedicalization: technoscientific transformations of the health, illness and US biomedicine. *American Sociological Review*. 68 (April): 161–94.
Conrad, P. (2007) *The Medicalisation of Society: On the Transformation of Human Conditions into Treatable Disorders*. Baltimore, MD: Johns Hopkins University Press.
Coveney, C., Nerlich, B. and Martin, P. (2009) Modafinil in the media: Medicalisation, metaphors and the body. *Social Science and Medicine*. 68: 487–95.
Crossley, N. (2004) *Sleep, reflexive embodiment and social networks*. Paper presented at the first ESRC 'Sleep and Society' seminar, 3 December, University of Warwick.
Damasio, A. (2003) *Looking for Spinoza*. London: Vintage.
——(2000) *The Feeling of What Happens*. London: Vintage.
——(1994) *Descartes Error*. London: Picador.
De Mul, J. (1999) The Informatization of the Worldview, *Information, Communication and Society*. 2(1): 69–94.
Fuller, S. (2006) *The New Sociological Imagination*. London: Sage.
——(1999) Review essay; The information age. *Science, Technology and Human Values*. 24(1) (winter): 159–66.
Gabe, J. and Bury, M. (1996) Halcion nights: a sociological account of a medical controversy. *Sociology*. 45(1): 447–69.
Giddens, A. (1996) Out of place: The rise of the network society. *The Times Higher Education Supplement*, 13 December. Available at: http://www.timeshighereducation.co.uk/story.asp?sectioncode=6&storycode=161993 (accessed 15 February 2011).
——(1991) *Modernity and Self-Identity*. Cambridge: Polity Press.
Gleick, J. (2000) *Faster: The Acceleration of Just About Everything*. London: Abacus.
——(1987) *Chaos*. London: Penguin.
Hackett, E. J., Amsterdamska, O., Lynch, M. and Wajcman, J. (eds.) (2007) *The Handbook of Science and Technology Studies (Third Edition)*. Cambridge, MA: The MIT Press.
Hardy, M. (2001) "E-health": The Internet and the Transformation of Patients into Consumers and Producers of Health Knowledge. *Information, Communication and Society*. 4(3): 388–405.
Harvey, D. (1989) *The Condition of Postmodernity*. Cambridge, MA: Blackwell.

Jessop, B. (2003) Informational capitalism and empire. *Source Studies in Political Economy*. 71–72: 39–58.

Jewson, N. D. (1976) The Disappearance of the Sick Man from Medical Cosmology 1770–1870. *Sociology*. 10(2): 225–44.

Kroll-Smith, S. (2003) Popular media and 'excessive daytime sleepiness': a study of rhetorical authority in medical sociology. *Sociology of Health and Illness*. 25: 625–43.

Lash, S. (2002) *Critique of Information*. London: Sage.

Marcuse, P. (2002) Depoliticizing globalization: The information age and the network society of Manuel Castells, in J. Eade and C. Mele (eds) *Investigating the City*. Oxford: Blackwell.

McLennan, G. (2003) Sociology's complexity. *Sociology*. 37(3): 547–64.

Mental Health Foundation (2011) *Sleep Matters*. Available at: http://www.mentalhealth.org.uk/our-work/campaigns/current-campaigns/sleep/ (accessed 18 April 2011).

Miah, A. and Rich, E. (2007) *The Medicalisation of Cyberspace*. London: Routledge.

Mills, C. W. (1959) *The Sociological Imagination*. New York: Oxford University Press.

Monaghan, L. and Williams, S. J. (in press) Stigma, in J. Gabe and L. Monaghan (eds.) *Key Concepts in Medical Sociology*, second edition. London: Sage.

Monge, P. R. and Contractor, N. S. (2003) *Theories of Communication Networks*. Oxford: Oxford University Press.

Moynihan R. and Cassells, A. (2005) *Selling Sickness: How The World's Biggest Pharmaceutical Companies Are Turning Us All Into Patients*. New York: Avalon Publishing Group Inc.

Nettleton, S. (2004) The emergence of e-scaped medicine? *Sociology*. 38(4): 661–79.

Nettleton, S., Burrows, R. and O'Malley, L. (2005) The mundane realities of the everyday use of the internet for health and their consequences for media convergence. *Sociology of Health and Illness*. 25(6): 589–607.

Osborne, T. and Rose, N. (2008) Editors' introduction: Revisiting British Sociology. *Sociological Review*. 56(4): 519–34.

Rose, N. (2007) *The Politics of Life Itself*. Princeton, NJ: Princeton University Press.

Savage, M. and Burrows, R. (2007) The coming crisis of empirical sociology. *Sociology*. 41(5): 885–99.

Scambler, G. (2009) Health-related stigma. *Sociology of Health and Illness*. 31: 441–55.

Seale, C. (2003) *Media and Health*. London: Sage.

Seale, C., Boden, S., Williams, S. J., Lowe, P. and Steinberg, D. L. (2007) Media constructions of sleep and sleep disorders: A study of UK national newspapers. *Social Science and Medicine*. 65: 418–30.

Stalder, F. (2006) *Manuel Castells*. Cambridge: Polity Press.

Tomlinson, J. (2007) *The Culture of Speed: The Coming of Immediacy*. London: Sage.

Urry, J. (2003) *Global Complexity*. Cambridge: Polity.

——(2000) Mobile Sociology. *British Journal of Sociology*. 51(1): 185–203.

Van Dijk, J. (1999) The one-dimensional network society of Manuel Castells. *Chronicle World*. Available at: http://www.chronicleworld.org (accessed 18 April 2011).

Virilio, P. (1986/1977) *Speed and Politics: An Essay on Dromology*. New York: Semiotext(e).

Waldby, C. (2000) *The Visible Human Project*. London: Routledge.

Wasserman, S. and Faust, K. (1994) *Social Network Analysis: Methods and Applications*. Cambridge: Cambridge University Press.

Watts, D. (2003) *Six Degrees: The Science of a Connected Age*. New York: W. W. Norton.

Webster, A. (2002) Innovative Health Technologies and the Social: Redefining Health, Medicine and the Body. *Current Sociology*. 50(3): 443–57.

Webster, F. (2002) *Theories of the Information Society*, second edition. New York: Routledge.

Webster, F. and Dimitriou, B. (eds) (2004) *Manuel Castells*, 3 vols. Thousand Oaks, CA: Sage.

Weisgerber, C. (2004) Turning to the internet for help on sensitive medical problems: A qualitative study of the construction of a sleep disorder through online interaction. *Information, Communication and Society*. 7: 554–74.

Westen, D. (2007) *The Political Brain*. New York: Public Affairs.

Widerberg, K. (2006) Embodying modern times: Investigating tiredness. *Time and Society*. 15(1): 105–20.

Williams, S. J. (2011) *The Politics of Sleep: Governing (Un)Consciousness in the Late Modern Age*. Basingstoke: Palgrave Macmillan.

——(2005) *Sleep and Society: Sociological Ventures into the (Un)Known*. London: Routledge.

——(2002) Sleep and health: reflections on the dormant society. *Health*. 6(2): 173–200.

Williams, S. J. and Bendelow, G. (1998) *The Lived Body*. London: Routledge.

Williams, S. J. and Crossley, N. (2008) Introduction: Sleeping bodies. *Body and Society*. 14: 1–15.

Williams, S. J., Seale, C., Boden, S., Lowe, P. and Steinberg, D. L. (2009) Waking Up to Sleepiness: Modafinil, the Media and the Pharmaceuticalisation of Everday/Night Life. In S. J. Williams, J. Gabe and P.B. Davis. *Pharmaceuticals and Society: Critical Discourses and Debates*. Oxford: Wiley-Blackwell.

——(2008) Medicalisation and beyond: The social construction of insomnia and snoring in the news. *Health*. 12(2): 251–68.

Wolf-Meyer, M. (2008) Sleep, signification and the abstract body of allopathic medicine. *Body 114*.

Woloshin, S. and Schwartz, L. M. (2006) Giving legs to restless legs: A case study of how the media help make people sick. *Public Library of Science – Medicine*. 3(4) (April): 170–78.

Index

Please note that page numbers relating to Notes will have the letter 'n' following the page number.

Abu-Lughod, J., 120
academia, 75
accelerated model, epidemiological transition theory, 114
adaptability, 171
agency, 9, 21, 79, 131; embodied, 96, 99; exceptional, transformational power of, 145; and structure, 134–5
Agricultural Revolution, 113
Akerstrom-Andersen, N., 58, 68n
Allsop, J., 42
Althusser, Louis, 169
always/might be (first-order form), 59
Amsterdam Project, neo-Gramscian perspective, 139
analytics (Luhmann), 55, 56–8, 61
Andersen, N. A., 56, 61
Angus, J., 76
anorexia, 156, 161
Anti-Oedipus (Deleuze and Guattari), 152, 159
anti-psychiatry, 41, 152
arche-health, 162, 163
Archer, Margaret, 79, 146, 147; and critical realism, 131–4, 145; ideal types of, 136–8; *Making our Way through the World*, 136, 138; *Structure, Agency and the Internal Conversation*, 135–6
Armelagos, G., 106
Armstrong, David, 10–11, 28
assemblages, 151, 154–6; contagious, 160; health/health care, 155–6, 162; hypochondriac, 161–2; neoplastic, 160; weight-loss, 161
Atkinson, W., 29
autonomous reflexives, 136, 137; and CEC/PE, 142–5; focused, 143, 144–5, 146, 147

autopoiesis/autopoietic systems, 50, 51, 68n
avoid/stop (second-order form), 62, 63

Batten disease, field of, 80–3
Baudrillard, Jean, 17, 21
Bauman, Zygmunt, 9, 20–31; fitness and health, 25–9; freedom and consumption, 20–2; liquid modernity, 20, 26, 29, 30; as 'prophet of postmodernity,' 29; regimentation of society, 23–4; society of consumers, shift to, 21, 22–5, 27; uncertainty, 23, 24, 26, 27–8, 29
Beck, Ulrich, 9, 12, 29, 30
Behague, D. P., 76
being-in-the-world, 96
Bell, Daniel, 170
Bentham, Jeremy, 8, 23, 24
Bhaskar, Roy, 131, 132, 133, 134, 145
binary code, 54
binary oppositions, 52, 57
biobanks, 11
biological citizenship, 13
biological knowledge, 14
biomedicine/biomedical imperialism, 10, 15, 37, 44, 159
bio-politics, 15, 98
bio-power, 8, 14, 15
Birth of the Clinic: An Archaeology of Medical Perception (Foucault), 8, 14, 89
Black Death, 113, 119, 120
blame, 143
Bobadilla, J. L., 127
bodily hexis, 73, 76–7, 84

194 Index

body: absence from everyday experience, 87; assemblages, 154–6, 160–2; Bauman on, 26; biological and social, 150, 153; body-with-organs (organism), 151, 153, 158–9; body-without-organs *see* body-without-organs (BwO); capacity to affect and be affected, 162, 164; creative force motivating, 153; death of *see* death; Deleuze and Guattari on, 150–66; embodied medical practice, 100–1; embodiment, phenomenology of, 91–3; five key properties, 88–9; flesh and blood, 88–91; Foucault on, 8, 9–10; habitus and bodily hexis, 73, 76–7; illness and bodily dys-appearance, 87, 98–100; lived, 92, 102; medical, 94–5; Merleau-Ponty on, 87–103; modern ideal of, 26; normal and abnormal, 15, 25, 27; reflexivity and bodily blind spot, 96–8; standardised, 23; as subject and relative entity, 10; territories of, 156–8; as tool or instrument, 92–3; what it can do (Deleuzian question), 151, 159–62, 163, 164
Body & Society, The (journal), 9
Body and Society (Turner), 88
body fat, 28–9
body mass index (BMI), 11
body-with-organs (organism), 151, 153, 158–9
body-without-organs (BwO), 151, 153–4, 157, 160, 161, 162, 163, 164
Boiko, Olga, 49–70, 57
Bourdieu, Pierre, 17, 29, 71–86; Batten disease, field of, 80–3; capital, 71, 72–4, 79–81, 84; criticisms of work, 79; field, 71, 72–4, 75, 79–83, 84; habitus, 71, 73, 74–7, 79, 83, 84, 139; lifeworld, 71–86; structure/agency debate, 71, 77–9; subjectivism/objectivism, 77, 78, 79
Braudel, Fernand, 104
Bretton Woods system, 139
Brown, P., 42
Buchanan, I., 161, 162, 163
bulk goods exchange network (BGN), 119, 120
Bunton, Robin, 11, 12
bureaucracies, 39, 41, 44

Canguilhem, G., 99–100
capital (Bourdieu), 71, 79–81, 84; and field, 72–4

capitalism, 113, 139–40, 142; informational, 171, 173, 185
capitalist-executive cabal (CEC), 139–41
cardiovascular diseases, 113
Cardoso, Fernando, 104
Care of the Self, The (Foucault), 8–9
Carroll, W., 139
Cartesian dualism, 88–91, 94
Castel, Robert, 12
Castells, Manuel, 167–92; academic posts, 168–9; appraising, 177–80; awards, honours and accolades, 169, 188; *Communication Power*, 168, 176; *Information Age, The*, 168; network society *see* network society; new social movements, 172–3; *Power of Identity, The*, 172; pre-eminence of morphology over action in work of, 179; on theory, 169
category error (Descartes), 91, 94, 101
CEC (capitalist-executive cabal), 139–41; and autonomous reflexivity, 142–5
certainty, 91; *see also* uncertainty
chains of communication, 52, 53
Chase-Dunn, C., 118, 120
Chew, S. C., 118
China, 105
choices, health behaviours, 74, 75, 78, 79
chronic diseases, 113
civil society, 55
Clarke, A., 189n
class, 21, 30
classic Western model, epidemiological transition theory, *108–12*, 114, 115
coercion, 172
cognitive insurance, 144
colonization: and medicalisation, 39–40; new social movements against, 41–3; and resistance in public health services, 44–6; social and health policy, 39
Coming of Post-industrial Society, The (Bell), 170
commitment, total, 144
commodification, 40, 45
commodity concentration index (CCI), 121, 122, 123
communication: and meaning, 57; real time, 58, 59
communication chains, 52, 53
communication power, 167, 169, 172, 183
Communication Power (Castells), 168, 176
communicative interaction, 35, 36, 37, 39, 44
communicative reflexives, 136, 137, 138
complexity theory, 174–5
composite units, 118

concentration index, *124*
concepts, 52
conformity, 24
Congo region, 125
connectivity, 59
Conrad, P., 189n
consciousness, 57, 77; false, 78, 145; Merleau-Ponty, 90, 92, 95, 96, 97, 98, 102n
constructionism, 88, 99
consumers: 'failed,' 21, 22; growth of consumerism and postmodernisation of society, 20; shift to society of, 21, 22–5, 27
consumption, and freedom, 20–2
contagious assemblage, 160
contextual incongruity, 146
contradiction, neo-Marxist notions, 131
Cook, I. G., 127
Corea, Gena, 10
core areas, 104–5, 117
cosmetic surgery, 10
critical realism, Archer on, 131–4, 145
Crossley, Nick, 87–103, 187
cross-national studies, 105
cultural capital, 72, 73, 81–2
cultural impoverishment, 39
culture, and lifeworld, 34
Currier, D., 164

Damasio, A., 189n
Dean, Mitchell, 9
death, 93, 94; main causes, 107, 113, 114, 121, 123
dedicated meta-reflexives, 146, 148
delayed model, epidemiological transition theory, 114, 115
Deleuze, Gilles, 17, 150–66; assemblages, 151, 154–6; and body, 151–3; body-with-organs (organism), 151, 153, 158–9; body-without-organs, 151, 153–4, 157, 160, 161, 163, 164; and health, 162–4; partnership with Guattari, 150, 151–2; publications by, 151, 152, 159; territorialisation, 151, 156–8, 159, 161, 164
Dement, William C., 181
De Mul, J., 185
dentine hypersensitivity case study (second-order forms), 59–60; avoid/stop, 62, 63; difference/change, 66; help/cure, 65; sharp/short pain, 60–2, 67; tolerate/accept, 63
dentist-patient communications, 59

dentists, 57
dependency theory, 104, 117
de Possas, A., 127
Descartes, René, 99; Cartesian dualism, 88–91, 94; error of, 91, 94, 101; external perspective on body, 92, 93; *Meditations*, 89, 91
desire, 152
determinism, 171, 178
deterritorialisation, 157, 159, 160, 162, 165
development theory, 117
Diagnostic and Statistical Manual of Mental Disorders (DSN), 14
Difference and Repetition (Deleuze), 151
difference/change (second-order form), 66
differentiation, 22, 50, 55
direct-to-consumer advertising, 17
disability, 15–16, 77, 84
disciplinary power, 8
Discipline and Punish (Foucault), 8, 24
disease: Batten disease, 80–3; cardiovascular, 113; and causes of death, 107, 113; chronic, 113; and dependency, 121–3; imagery of, and eugenics, 22; impact of world system on, in West Africa, 123–6; infectious, 107, 113, 119, 120; *see also* illness
disenchantment, 35
distinctions, 52
distorted communication, 36
doctor-patient interaction, 36, 57
Dorling, Daniel, 146
Douglas, Mary, 11
doxic habitus, 74, 78; non-doxic field, 75, 84
Duff, C., 163
Dummer, T. J. B., 127
durable inequality, 30
Durkheim, D. E., 95

Eagleton, Terry, 147
eating disorders, 156, 161
Ecolé de Hautes en Science Sociales (Paris), 168
economic capital, 72, 73, 81
Economy and Society (Weber), 178
Edwards, Gemma, 33–48
embodiment: character of, 164; embodied agency, 96, 99; embodied health movements, 42, 43; embodied medical practice, 100–1; embodied nature of habitus, 76; health as embodied phenomenon, 150; phenomenology of, 91–3; territorialisation, 157, 157–8; *see also* body
Engels, Friedrich, 145

entangled hierarchy, 61
environmental breast cancer movement, US, 42, 43
environmental social movements, 43
epidemiological polarization, 126
epidemiological transition theory (ETT), 106–16; accelerated model, 114; ambiguity, 106, 107; classic Western model, *108–12*, 114, 115; delayed model, 114, 115; models of epidemiological transition, 114–15; propositions, 107; stages, 107, 112; state-centrism of, 105, 116; and world system theory, 105–6, 117–18, 121, 126
epistemic fallacy, 132, 135
Epworth Sleepiness Scale (ESS), 184
e-scaping, 185, 186
ethology, 163
Euro-dollar, 139
excessive daytime sleepiness (EDS), 184, 185
exclusion, 173
existence, in phenomenology, 92
expert perspective, and modern medicine, 36–8
explanatory methodology (EM), 132
Expressionism in Philosophy: Spinoza (Deleuze and Guattari), 151
external zone, 120, 121
eyesight, 97–8

failed consumers, 21, 22
false consciousness, 78, 145
fat, 28–9
Featherstone, Mike, 9
feminism, 10, 93
Fernand Braudel Centre, 105
fertility, 114
field (Bourdieu), 71, 75, 79–80; Batten disease, 80–3; and capital, 72–4; entering and exiting, 81, 84; non-doxic, 75, 84
financialization, 139
first-order forms, 58, 60, 62, 63, 65
fitness and health, 25–9; whether fitness a new dimension of health, 29–31
Fitzpatrick, R., 113
flesh and blood, 88–91
flexibility, 171, 174
fly in the ointment metaphor, 25–6
focused autonomous reflexives, 143, 146, 147; six core constituents, 144–5
Forbes, A., 75
form analysis, 57, 67; and dentine hypersensitivity *see* dentine

hypersensitivity case study (second-order forms); first-order forms, 58, 60, 62, 63, 65; objects, 58; second-order forms, 58, 62–6; semantic forms, 59
Foucault, Michel, 7–19, 23, 88; application of concepts, 9; biological citizenship, 13; *Birth of the Clinic: An Archaeology of Medical Perception*, 8, 14, 89; blindspots in work of, 16; body, 8, 9–10; disability discourses, 15–16; discourse, 8; 'early' and 'later' work of, 8; 'Foucault effect,' 7, 17; governmentality, 10, 11, 12, 16; and language use, 16; limitations of work/related scholarship, 16–17; power-knowledge, 8, 10; practices of health and medicine, 13–15; public health and risk, 10–12; technologies of the self, 9, 11, 16; as theorist, 7–9; 'toolkit' of ideas offered by, 7, 17
fourth world, 173
Fox, Nick J., 14, 64, 150–66, 151–66, 162, 163
fractured reflexives, 136, 138, 148
Fredriksen, S., 37
freedom, and consumption, 20–2
Freedom (Bauman), 21
Frenk, J., 127
Freud, Sigmund, 152
FTSE, 142
Fuller, S., 179
functional necessity, 45
functional structural theory, 50
fundamentalist ideology, 144

Galileo, 89, 91
Garland, D., 16
GBH ('greedy bastards hypothesis'), 138, 139, 142, 143, 145, 147
Gellner, E., 132
gender and health, 10
genealogy, 8
genetic structuralism, 77
genetic testing, 10
Gibson, Barry, 49–70
Giddens, Anthony, 9, 12, 21, 29, 30, 178
global elite, 179
goods-purveyors, individuals as, 25
governmentality, 10, 11, 12, 16
grand theory, 16
gravity, 156
Great British Sleep Survey, 181
grief counselling, 37

Guattari, Felix, 150–66; assemblages, 151, 154–6; and body, 151–3; body-with-organs (organism), 151, 153, 158–9; body-without-organs, 151, 153–4, 157, 160, 161, 162, 163, 164; and health, 162–4; partnership with Deleuze, 150, 151–2; publications by, 151, 152, 159; territorialisation, 151, 156–8, 159, 161, 164
Gunder Frank, Andre, 104

Habermas, Jürgen, 33–48, 138, 143, 147; colonization, 39–40, 41–3, 44–6; communicative interaction, 35, 36, 37, 39, 44; expert perspective, and modern medicine, 36–8; lifeworld, 33, 38–41, 43, 44–6; patient perspective, everyday health, 34–6; rationalization, 35, 37, 38, 44; social movements, new, 33, 41–3; state bureaucracies, 39, 41, 44; system, 33–4, 36–8, 43, 44–6; taken for grantedness, 35
habit, 100
habit/lifestyle (second-order form), 64–5
habitus, 71, 73, 74–6, 79, 83, 84, 139; and bodily hexis, 73, 76–7; embodied nature, 76; *see also* reflexivity
Hacking, Ian, 13
Hall, T., 118, 120
Harper, K., 106
health and medicine: capacity of body to affect and be affected, 162, 164; collective action around, 41–3; fitness and health, 25–9; Foucault on, 7–19; illness vs. health, 162–3; modern medicine and expert perspective, 36–8; politics and morality in, 33–48; practices of, 13–15; sleep and health, 180–8; *see also* body; disease; illness
health consumer groups, 42
health identity, paradox of, 64
health/illness (second-order form), 58
health inequalities, sociology of, 131–49; capitalist-executive cabal, 139–41; GBH ('greedy bastards hypothesis'), 138, 139, 142, 143, 145, 147; ideology, 145; resistance, 145–7; state power elite, 141–2
Heidegger, Martin, 95, 102n
height, body, 97
help/cure (second-order form), 65
Herfindahl-Hirschmann index, *124*
Higgs, Paul, 20–31

High Pay Commission, Interim Report, 142
History of Sexuality, The (Foucault), 8, 15
Hobbes, Thomas, 142
holism, 94, 95
homo sacer, 28
human flourishing, 27
human subject, 13
Husserl, Edmund, 89–90, 91–2, 95, 102n
Hyde, A., 45
Hyde, Martin, 104–30
hydrogenated fat, 28
hypochondriac assemblage, 161–2

iatrogenesis, social and cultural, 27
ideal types (Archer), 136–8
ideal types (Castells), 173
identity, 173
ideology, 145; fundamentalist, 144
Illich, Ivan, 27
illness: Bauman on, 29; and bodily dys-appearance, 87, 98–100; doctor-patient interaction, 36; and fitness, 27–8, 29; vs. health, 162–3; living with, 71; personal experience of, 34; *see also* disease; health and medicine
illusion, 78
impairment, vs. disability, 15
imperative of health, 28
imperialism, 104
indeterminacy of fitness, 31
India, 105
individualisation, 26, 29
industrial capital, 139–40
Industrial Revolution, 113
infectious diseases, 107, 113, 119, 120
influenza, 119
information age, 167, 169, 170, 181
Information Age, The (Castells), 168, 170
informational capitalism, 171, 173, 185
informationalism, 169, 171, 172
informational politics, 173
informational society, 171
information and communication technologies (ICTs), 168, 171–2
information exchange network (IN), 119–20
inner speech/inner reflexive dialogue, 135, 136, 137, 147
institutionalised inequality, 30
instrumental action, 37
instrumental rationality, 35, 37, 38
intellectual debts, 168–9, 185
intellectual property, 179
intentionality, 90, 93, 97
intermittent pain, 61

internal conversation, 135, 147
International Classifications of Diseases (ICD), 14
intransitivity/intransitive entities, 132
Iraq war, 177

Japan, 114, 135
Jenkins, R., 71, 77, 78, 79
Jewson, N. D., 185
Journal of World-Systems Research, 105
juridification, 39, 44, 45

Kelleher, D., 43
King, M., 51, 68n
Kroll-Smith, S., 184, 185

Lacan, Jacques, 152
Lagos, Africa, 125
language, 157
Laws of Form (Spencer-Brown), 52
Leder, D., 87, 96, 98, 99
legitimising identity, 173
life expectancies, 107, 113, 115
Life Exposed: Biological Citizens After Chernobyl (Petryna), 13
Life in Fragments (Bauman), 26
lifestyle, 64–5; illnesses, 113
lifeworld, 43, 44–6, 80, 102n; conflict with system, 33–4, 38–41, 57; impact of health and illness on, 71–86; patient perspective, everyday health, 34–6; voice of, 35, 36, 38, 40
lifeworld detachment, 144
line of flight, 160
lines of flight, 158, 159
Liquid Life (Bauman), 26
liquid modernity (Bauman), 20, 26, 29, 30
lived body, 92, 102
Logic of Sense, The (Deleuze), 151
look/feel (semantic form), 59
Luhmann, Niklas, 49–70; analytics of, 55, 56–8, 61; application of ideas to study of health and illness, 53–5; dentine hypersensitivity *see* dentine hypersensitivity case study (second-order forms); form analysis, 58–9, 62–6, 67; on Parsons, 50, 51; Pelikan on, 53–5, 56; sensitivity pain, 60–2; social systems theory, 49–55, 57, 58, 67; theory pieces, 49, 50
Luhmann Explained: From Souls to Systems (Moeller), 68n
Lumme-Sandt, K., 76
Lupton, Deborah, 11–12

Machiavelli, Niccolò, 143
Mackenbach, J. P., 107
magnetic resonance imaging (MRI), 10
Making our Way through the World (Archer), 136, 138
Marcuse, P., 179
marginalisation of the other, 21, 30
market principles, 37
Marmot Report (2010), 138, 146
Marx, Karl, 77, 78, 178
Marxism, 9, 16, 17, 104; structural, 169, 170, 172
mass media, 21–2
mass self-communication, 186
maternity care, 45
matter, 88, 91, 92
Maturana, Humberta, 50
Mauss, Marcel, 92
McDonnell, O., 73
McKeown, T., 114
McNeill, W., 120
Mead, G. H., 95, 97
meaning, 172
medical body, 94–5
medical gaze, 14, 94
medicalisation, 27, 31, 40, 186
medical knowledge, 185
medical professional/patient (second-order form), 58
Meditations (Descartes), 89, 91
Mental Health Foundation, 181
Merleau-Ponty, Maurice: on body, 87–103; consciousness, 90, 92, 95, 96, 97, 98, 102n; embodied agency, 96, 99; embodied medical practice, 100–1; embodiment, phenomenology of, 91–3; flesh and blood, 88–91; illness and bodily dys-appearance, 87, 98–100; medical body, 94–5; perception/perceptual experiences, 87, 89, 90, 92, 93; perspective, 96, 97–8, 101; *Phenomenology of Perception, The*, 96; reflexivity and bodily blind spot, 87, 96–8; science and philosophy, 95–6; *Structure of Behaviour, The*, 95, 96; vantage point, 92, 98
meta-effort, 24
meta-reflexives, 136, 137, 138; dedicated, 146, 148
Metro Naps, 187
metropoles (core areas), 104–5, 117
Michailakis, D., 63, 64–5
micro-political life politics, 137, 141
Mills, C. W., 183

minds, 89, 99, 176–7
Mingers, John, 68n
minimum standard of living, 25
Mishler, E., 35
mobile information technologies, 184
Modafinil, 184
modernisation theory, 104, 115, 117
Modernity and the Holocaust (Bauman), 20, 22
modes of production, 170
Moeller, H.-G., 51, 68n
money capital concept, 139
morality, and politics, 33–48
morphogenesis, 132, 134–5, 148
morphogenetic structures, 134
morphostatic actions, 134

napping pods, 187
National Health Service (NHS), UK, 45, 75, 142
nationality, 156
National Sleep Foundation (NSF), US, 187
nation-state, role, 22, 23
neo-liberalism, 12, 17, 139, 145
Neolithic revolution, 112
neoplastic assemblage, 160
Neruda, Pablo, 146
Nettleton, S., 185
network society, 169, 170–7, 179–80; informational capitalism, 171, 173, 185; mind, 176–7; networks, 73, 174–5; nodes, 174; organisation, 174–6; production, 170–2; sleep and health in, 180–8; space of flows, 175; technology, 170–1
network state, 173
neuroscience, 177
'neuro' turn, 176
new genetics, 13
new social movements, 33, 41–3, 172–3
Newton, P. D., 79
Nietzsche, Friedrich, 152
Nietzschean instinct, 144
Niger Delta, 126
Nigerian Civil War (1967–70), 125
nomadology, 159
normal and abnormal body, 15, 25, 27
normalisation, 11
Novas, Carlos, 13

obesity, 11
objectification of objectification, 75
objectivism/subjectivism (Bourdieu), 77, 78, 79
objects, 58

Oborne, P., 141
Offe, C., 44, 45
Olszynko-Gryn, J., 106–7, 114
Omran, Abdel, 106–16, 121, 123
ontology, 132; social, 132, 133
oppression, gender-based, 10
order, 23
organisation, 174–6
organism (body-with-organs), 151, 153, 158–9

pain *see* dentine hypersensitivity case study; sensitivity pain
Panopticon, 8, 23, 24
paradox of difference, 66, 67
parental capital, 82
Parsons, Talcott, 28, 50, 51, 57
participant objectification, 75
pastoral power, 14
patient activism, 13
patient-centred medicine, 14
patient perspective, everyday health, 34–6
patients, as 'clients' of health services, 41
patriotism, 177
Pearson's correlation coefficients, 127n
Pelikan, J., 53–5, 56, 66, 67
perception/perceptual experiences, 87, 89, 90, 92, 93
peripheral areas, 105, 117
personality, and lifeworld, 34
perspective: Bourdieu, 76–7; expert, 36–8; Foucault, 12, 14, 15; Habermas, 34–8; Luhmann, 50, 53, 55, 57, 58, 62, 67, 68n; Merleau-Ponty, 96, 97–8, 101; patient, 34–6
Petersen, Alan, 7–19
Petryna, Adriana, 13
phenomenology, of embodiment, 91–3
Phenomenology of Perception, The (Merleau-Ponty), 96
philosophy, and science, 95–6
physical capital, 73, 81, 82
Pickett, Kate E., 146
places, space of, 175
political activism, 42
Political Anatomy of the Body (Armstrong), 10
political class, 141
political/military exchange network (PMN), 119, 120
Political Theory in the Welfare State (Luhmann), 51
politics: experience, 172; identity, 173; and morality, 33–48; power, 172
Pompeii, 135

population health, 105
Porpora, D., 134
positive difference/change (second-order form), 66
positivism, 132
postmodernism, 20, 29, 134
Potts, A., 163
power: of agency, 145; bio-power, 8, 14, 15; Castells on, 167, 169, 172; communication, 167, 169, 172, 183; disciplinary, 8; Foucault on, 8, 10, 14; network society, 177; pastoral, 14; sovereign, 8; surgical, 14; will-to-power, 152
power elite (PE), state, 141–2; and autonomous reflexivity, 142–5
power-knowledge, 8, 10
Power of Identity, The (Castells), 172
power relationships, 177
practical social theories (PST), 132
prestige good exchange network (PGN), 119, 120
Prince, The (Machiavelli), 143
privatisation, 24
producers, society of: shift to society of consumers, 21, 22–5, 27
production, network society, 170–2
productive capital concept, 139
project identity, 173
psychiatry, 37
psychoanalysis, 152
public health: binary code for, 54; vs. clinical medicine, 55; colonization and resistance in public health services, 44–6; experts, 54–5; and risk, 10–12

quality of care, 76
quality of life, 31

rationalization, 35, 37, 38, 44, 137
realism, critical, 131–4, 145
reductionism, biomedical perspectives, 15
reflexivity, 97, 135–8; autonomous *see* autonomous reflexives; and bodily blind spot, 87, 96–8; Bourdieu on, 71, 75, 79, 83; communicative reflexives, 136, 137, 138; fractured reflexives, 136, 138, 148; meta-reflexives, 136, 137, 138, 146, 148; *see also* habitus
regimentation of society, 23–4
religion, 133
repetition, 59
resistance, 16, 145–7, 152, 159, 164
resistance identity, 173

resource dependency, 141
restless legs syndrome, 183
reterritorialisation, 157, 158
risk, and public health, 10–12
Risk Society, The (Beck), 12
Roche-Reid, B., 45
Rose, Nicholas, 9, 13
Rosie, Anthony, 104–30
Ryle, Gilbert, 91, 94

Sartre, Jean-Paul, 92, 102n
saturated fat, 28
Sawicki, Jana, 10
Scambler, Graham, 43, 131–49
Scambler, Sasha, 71–86
Schirmer, W., 63, 64–5
schizoanalysis, 159
science and philosophy, 95–6
science and technology, 170, 189n
second-order distinctions, 52–3
second-order forms, 58, 62–6, 65
sedentism, 112–13
self-determination, 9
self-formation regime, 24
self-help groups, 41, 42
semantics, 59
semi-peripheral areas, 104, 105
Sennett, Richard, 29
sensation, 25, 90
sensitive toothpastes, 59–60, 65–6, 67
sensitivity pain, 60–2
Sensodyne, 65
Shakespeare, Tom, 15
sharp/short pain (second-order form), 60–2, 67
Shen, C., 115–16, 121
sleep, and health, 167, 180–8; in information age, 183–6; sleep industry, 186–8; social arrhythmia, 183; timeless time, 181–3
sleep laboratory/clinic, 183
sleep paralysis, 184
Smith, Dennis, 29
Smith, M., 141–2
social arrhythmia, 182, 183
social capital, 72–3, 81, 82
social class, 21, 30
social constructionism, 88
socialisation, 74, 84
Social Meaning of Surgery, The (Fox), 14
social movements: new, 33, 41–3, 172–3; old, 41
social ontology (SO), 132, 133

social relations, 170
social systems theory (Luhmann), 49–53, 57, 58, 67; application to the study of health and illness, 53–5
society: and lifeworld, 34; morphogenetic nature, 132; as open system, 131–2; of producers, shift to society of consumers, 21, 22–5, 27; terminology, 118
socio-cultural interaction, 134
socio-economic change, 114
socio-economic classifications (SECs), 138, 146
Sociological Imagination (Mills), 183
sociological renewal, 188
sociology of health inequalities *see* health inequalities, sociology of
sovereign power, 8
Soviet statism, 189n
space of flows, 175, 181
space of places, 175
Spencer-Brown, G., 49, 52
Spinoza, Baruch, 151
Stalder, F., 170, 172, 174, 175, 179, 181, 182, 189n
standardised body, 23
state bureaucracies, 39, 41, 44
state philosophy, 151
Steverding, D., 125
stratified reality, 133
structural conditioning, 134
structural determinism, 131, 147
structural functionalism, 50, 51
structural Marxism, 169, 170, 172
structure, 74, 78; and agency, 134–5; structure/agency debate, 71, 77–9
Structure, Agency and the Internal Conversation (Archer), 135–6
Structure of Behaviour, The (Merleau-Ponty), 95, 96
subjectivism/objectivism (Bourdieu), 77, 78, 79
substances, 88, 89, 90, 91, 94
surgical power, 14
surveillance, 25; of body, 10
surveillance cameras, 8
surveillance medicine, 28
symbolically generalised media, 57–8
symbolic capital, 73, 78, 81, 82
symbolic violence, 78
system, 43, 44–6; conflict with lifeworld, 33–4, 38–41, 57; as modern medicine and expert perspective, 36–8
Systems, not people, make society happen (King), 68n

taken for grantedness, 7, 8, 35, 94, 98, 99
tallness, 97
technologies of the self (Foucault), 9, 11, 16
technology, network society, 170–1
technosocial world, 170
territorialisation, 151, 159, 161, 164
Theory of Social Practice and Society (Bourdieu), 77
theory pieces (Luhmann), 49, 50
Thompson, J. B., 79
Thousand Plateaus, A (Deleuze and Guattari), 152
Tilly, C., 30
time: real time, 58, 59; simultaneous, 175; as socially constructed, 77–8; timeless, 181–3
time-space compression, 185
tolerate/accept (second-order form), 63
toothpaste, sensitive, 59–60, 65–6, 67
Touraine, Alain, 168
trade dependency, 121–2
transfactuality, 132–3
transient pain, 61
treatment-seeking paradox, 66, 67
tunnel vision, 144
Turner, Brian, 88
Turner, Bryan, 9

uncertainty, 83; Bauman on, 23, 24, 26, 27–8, 29
underperformance, 27
Understanding Society project, 181
University of Sheffield, ethics committee, 60
unsaturated fat, 28
Use of Pleasure, The (Foucault), 8

vagrancy, 23
value rationality, 137
van Dijk, J., 179
vantage point, 92, 98
Varela, Francisco, 50
vertical power elite model, 141
Virschow, Rudolf, 145
Virtanen, P., 76
voice of lifeworld, 35, 36, 38, 40
voice of medicine, 36, 38, 40, 185
Vygotsky, L., 135

Wacquant, L. J. D., 72
Wainwright, S., 75, 78
Wallerstein, Immanuel, 104, 105, 116–17, 120, 127

Ward, K. J., 64, 163
war on terror, 177
Weber, Max, 35, 37, 137, 178
Webster, F., 185
weight gain or loss, 98
weight-loss assemblage, 161
Weisgerber, C., 184
Weisz, G., 106–7, 114
welfare policy, 22
welfare state, 31, 39
West Africa, 104, 105, 106;
  impact of world system on disease and death, 123–6
Westminster power elite model, 141
What is Philosophy? (Deleuze and Guattari), 152
Wieviorka, Michel, 188
Wiley, N., 136
Williams, Simon J., 73, 78–9, 81, 134–5, 167–92
Williamson, J. B., 115–16, 121
will-to-power, 152
women: low health habitus, 76; objectification of body, 93

Work, consumerism and the new poor (Bauman), 22
work ethic, 22
working classes, 21
World Congress of Sociology, 188
world system theory (WST), 104, 116–23;
  analysis categories, refining, 120–1;
  boundaries, 119; construction of world systems, 118–20; definitions, 116;
  dependency and disease, 121–3; and epidemiological transition theory, 105–6, 117–18, 121, 126; history of world-system, 105; West Africa, impact of world system on disease and death, 123–6
World Trade Organisation (WTO), 121, 122

xeno-transplantation, 10

Young, I., 93

Zimbabwe, 122

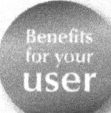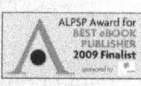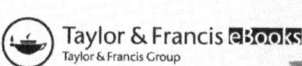

Lightning Source UK Ltd.
Milton Keynes UK
UKHW02f0813140218
317838UK00005B/200/P